THE DRUG TREATMENT
OF
TUBERCULOSIS

THE DRUG TREATMENT
OF
TUBERCULOSIS

By

ARCHIBALD C. COHEN, M.D.

Chief, Medical Service
Veterans Administration Hospital
Butler, Pennsylvania

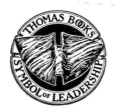

CHARLES C THOMAS • PUBLISHER
Springfield · Illinois · U. S. A.

Published and Distributed Throughout the World by
CHARLES C THOMAS · PUBLISHER
BANNERSTONE HOUSE
301-327 East Lawrence Avenue, Springfield, Illinois, U.S.A.
NATCHEZ PLANTATION HOUSE
735 North Atlantic Boulevard, Fort Lauderdale, Florida, U.S.A.

*With THOMAS BOOKS careful attention is given to all details of
manufacturing and design. It is the Publisher's desire to present books
that are satisfactory as to their physical qualities and artistic possibilities
and appropriate for their particular use. THOMAS BOOKS will be true
to those laws of quality that assure a good name and good will.*

Printed in the United States of America
H-13

To my wife,

Shulamith Rabb Cohen,

who stimulated me to begin this book,
encouraged me to complete it, and has
been my constant adviser and helper
during its preparation

PREFACE

In the past two decades the character of tuberculosis has changed more than in all previous history. The death rate has dropped spectacularly, the duration of disability has become shorter, treatment is usually successful, relapses are few, collapse therapy has almost entirely disappeared, and resectional surgery has become both safer and less necessary. Effective drugs have brought about these changes.

Since 1944, a considerable number of drugs have been discovered which are effective in preventing the growth and multiplication of M. tuberculosis. So good are these drugs that almost the only cause of treatment failure is inadequate treatment. In order to use them wisely, the physician must know a great deal about these drugs—their effectiveness and toxicity, the development of bacterial resistance, the best combinations, the optimum duration of treatment, the management of hypersensitivity and the situations which make resectional surgery desirable, to name a few matters. Internists and specialists in tuberculosis have this information, of course, but they are seldom the physicians who see the tuberculous patients first.

When the diagnosis of tuberculosis is made, many practical questions present themselves at once. Should the patient go to a hospital for treatment, or should he be treated at home? What drugs should be used, in what dosage, and for how long? Should the patient's household contacts receive any treatment? The physicians who make the initial diagnosis of tuberculosis and must take intelligent action to get effective treatment started are usually general practitioners or specialists in fields remote from pulmonary disease—orthopedic surgeons, urologists and pediatricians, for instance. For them this book is primarily written. It is hoped sincerely that this book will not only be of practical value to them in the care of these patients, but also that it will help to improve understanding of the new resources available for the treatment of this old disease.

Archibald C. Cohen

[vii]

ACKNOWLEDGMENTS

A BOOK OF this nature is never really the work of one person. In one way or another, many make a contribution. It is my privilege here to acknowledge some of the most important.

Several people were helpful in the preparation of the manuscript. Mrs. Ann Ovington typed several drafts and most of the final copy, and assisted with the proofreading. Mrs. Betty Atkinson helped to type the final copy of the manuscript. My wife's stylistic criticisms were always constructive and beneficial, and her assistance in proofreading was invaluable. The Medical Illustration Service of the Pittsburgh Veterans Administration Hospital prepared all the roentgenologic illustrations.

Miss Clare Heibel, Hospital Librarian, assisted by checking references, providing books and journals from the hospital library as needed, and borrowing books and journals from other libraries when they were not available locally.

Thanks are due to the members of the Tuberculosis Staff of the Butler Veterans Administration Hospital, whose many discussions on the management of tuberculosis helped to crystallize my own opinions.

Finally, I must acknowledge the great debt due to my patients who, in the final analysis, taught us all we know about the drug treatment of tuberculosis.

A.C.C.

CONTENTS

THE DRUG TREATMENT
OF
TUBERCULOSIS

Chapter I

HISTORICAL INTRODUCTION

T UBERCULOSIS HAS AFFLICTED mankind since early times, and has probably been its greatest scourge. It existed in the Egypt of the Pharaohs, was described as the "King of Diseases" in the Indian Vedas, and was common in Greece at the time of Hippocrates. Accurate records of its frequency and its mortality are not available until fairly recent times, but 30 per cent of all deaths in London in 1801 were due to tuberculosis, and 23 per cent of all deaths in New York City in 1804 were due to this disease. It is probable that throughout human history more people have died of tuberculosis than of any other single cause. Not only was it a major cause of death, but it was also an important cause of disability and pauperization.

Though tuberculosis was one of the most feared of human diseases, there was little that could be done about it until recently. The basis of treatment had long been rest and good nutrition, and in the twentieth century, collapse therapy was usually added. Rest was frequently strict and long continued. Collapse procedures were of many kinds, of which the most widely used were artificial pneumothorax, phrenic nerve paralysis, and thoracoplasty. Collapse procedures were designed to reduce the motion of the lungs, to close cavities, and to favor scarring of the lesion, but they were not notably successful.

Artificial pneumothorax was a relatively simple procedure, and once well established could be carried on at home or in out-patient clinics. However, it was necessary to continue giving refills for a number of years, there was usually serious damage to the pulmonary function, there were many complications (some of which were serious or even fatal), and worst of all, most patients were not benefited. Phrenic nerve paralysis was a simple procedure, relatively free of complications, but rather ineffective. Thoracoplasty was an operation done in several stages; it was deforming and usually unsuccessful. There were many other varieties of collapse therapy, such as pneumoperitoneum and oleothorax, and each of these had a vogue for a time, but these, too, caused many complications and were rather ineffective.

In 1938, Drolet made a statistical survey of the case fatality rates in a number of areas in the United States and in England and Wales, and found that there was no significant improvement over a period of twenty years, while the mortality had dropped by more than 50 per cent during these same years. From this, he drew the conclusion that the reduction in mortality rates was due to segregation of active cases and to improvement of living and working conditions, and that the treatment used at that time had little or no effect on the case fatality rates. Since the treatment of the 1930's—rest and collapse therapy—was now shown to be almost ineffective, the search for effective drugs was intensified.

Tuberculosis is an ancient disease, and the search for drugs and medications with which to treat it is almost as ancient as the disease itself. For a very long time people have dreamed of drugs which would influence the course of tuberculosis favorably, and hundreds have been tried. Until recently none of these have been specific. The hundreds of drugs which have found favor at one time or another have had either no value or only symptomatic value. Among those which have been used are creosote, guiacol, chaulmoogra oil and its derivatives, and a host of medications for the relief of fever, cough and night sweats, the control of hemorrhage and the improvement of appetite.

After Ehrlich's discovery that the azo dye trypan red was successful in trypanosomal infections and that organic arsenical compounds were effective in the treatment of syphilis, there was an acceleration of the search for drugs effective against tuberculosis. Many dyes were investigated, especially trypan red, trypan blue and methylene blue, alone and in combination with iodine, copper and mercury, but none had any therapeutic effect. Arsenic compounds were tried with equal lack of success. Copper compounds were used, both experimentally and clinically, and favorable results were reported in a number of cases from the use of cyanocuprol, but later studies failed to confirm this and these drugs were abandoned.

Mercury had been investigated by Koch as early as 1890, and by others in the 1920's, but without success. In the second and third decades of this century, gold compounds came into use. Sanocrysin (sodium gold thiosulfate)(1) (2), and krysolgan and solganal-B Oleosum (3) (complex gold compounds) were tried, and it was believed for a time that they stimulated the reticuloendothelial system and thereby increased resistance to tuberculosis. The toxicity of gold compounds was impressive, and carefully controlled studies failed to show that they benefited tuberculous patients, but they were used to a limited extent until the early 1940's. In spite of these numerous failures, Wells and Long wrote in 1932, "A specific chemotherapy of tuberculosis has not been found, and it may be long in coming . . . but it is not a closed chapter. . . . Probably success with other bacterial infection will be needed to stimulate a new attack on tuberculosis (4)." These words have proved to be prophetic.

In 1935, Domagk discovered that sulfonamides were effective in the treatment of experimental streptococcal infection (5). This led to the use of a number of sulfonamides in experimental tuberculosis. Sulfanilamide, sulfapyridine, sulfathiazol and sulfadiazine were tried and found wanting (6). These drugs have some tuberculostatic activity in the test tube and even in experimental animals, but the doses required are toxic doses and the improvement in animals is minimal, so the sulfonamide drugs were soon abandoned. However, they opened a line of investigation which has continued until the present time.

The sulfones next appeared on the therapeutic horizon. These drugs, chemically closely related to the sulfonamides, were first used in tuberculosis in 1937, and were found to be effective both in the test tube and in experimental animals. In the next ten years nearly a hundred compounds were prepared that were chemically related to the parent drug 4,4'-diaminodiphenylsulfone, and were tried in the test tube and in experimental animals. The most promising of these, promin, diasone, promizole and sulfetrone, also received clinical trial. It soon became clear that these drugs were valuable, and that for the first time chemotherapeutic agents were available which would help in the cure of experimental and clinical tuberculosis.

Promin was shown to have a suppressive action on tuberculosis in guinea pigs, reducing the number of bacilli in the lesions and actually sterilizing some of the lesions (7). However, eradication of the bacilli was not accomplished, so that when treatment was stopped the disease progressed again. In human tuberculosis, particularly when the disease was fresh and exudative in character, there was often a good clinical response, accompanied by x-ray clearing and even by conversion of the sputum. However, use for a brief period was ineffective, while long-term use often resulted in secondary anemia and sometimes caused agranulocytosis. Diasone proved to be almost ineffective (8). Promizole was found not to be particularly helpful in pulmonary tuberculosis, but it greatly prolonged survival in miliary and meningeal tuberculosis (9). It sometimes caused agranulocytosis, and it often caused goiter as a result of blocking the production of thyroxin. Sulfetrone arrived on the scene a little later, and, since streptomycin was already available, it did not receive as much study as the other sulfones. It was moderately successful in the treatment of pulmonary tuberculosis, but its toxic effects discouraged extensive investigation in man. It produced cyanosis, dyspnoea, anemia and goiter.

Sulfones are believed to act as antimetabolites. They are little used now, because they have been replaced by better drugs. However, they were encouraging. A great deal of work had been done with other drugs previously, over a period of several decades, and nothing worthwhile had been found. With the sulfones, for the first time, chemotherapeutic agents were available which did not offer symptomatic relief but attacked M. tuberculosis directly. Though these agents were too toxic for widespread use, and were effective to a limited extent only, this was a great step forward. Further work was done to prepare chemically related drugs, and this led, some years later, to the thiosemicarbazones. In the evaluation of the sulfones, techniques were worked out to permit the rapid evaluation of the effectiveness of new drugs against M. tuberculosis in experimental animals. Thus the sulfones prepared the way for the modern chemotherapy of tuberculosis, which began in 1944 with the discovery of streptomycin.

REFERENCES

1. MOLLGAARD, H.: *Chemotherapy of Tuberculosis, Nyt Nordisk Forlag,* Copenhagen, 1924.

2. AMBERSON, J. B., McMAHON, B. T., AND PINNER, M.: A clinical trial of sanocrysin in pulmonary tuberculosis, *Amer. Rev. Tuberc., 24:* 401, 1931.

3. SELIGSON, F.: Treatment with solganal-B Oleosum, *Amer. Rev. Tuberc., 43:*394, 1941.

4. WELLS, H. G., AND LONG, E. R.: *The Chemistry of Tuberculosis,* 2nd ed., Williams and Wilkins, 1932, p. 452.

5. DOMAGK, G.: Ein Beitrag zur Chemotherapie der Bakteriellen Infektionen, *Deutsche Med. Wschr., 61:*250, 1935.

6. FELDMAN, W. H., AND HINSHAW, H .C.: Sulfapyridine in experimental tuberculosis. *Amer. Rev. Tuberc., 41:*732, 1940.

7. FELDMAN, W. H., AND HINSHAW, H. C.: Promin in experimental tuberculosis (Effects of prolonged treatment with sodium). *Amer. Rev. Tuberc., 51:*268, 1945.

8. BENSON, L., AND GOODMAN, L.: Diasone therapy of pulmonary tuberculosis; its clinical efficacy and toxicity, *Amer. Rev. Tuberc. 51:*463, 1945.

9. MILGRAM, L., LEVITT, I., AND UNNA, M.: Promizole treatment of miliary tuberculosis; toxic effects on thyroid gland and maturation. *Amer. Rev. Tuberc., 55:*140, 1947.

Chapter II

THE PATHOGENESIS OF TUBERCULOSIS

THE MOST COMMON route by which tubercle bacilli enter the body is the respiratory tract. Far less commonly, bacilli establish their first infection in the intestinal tract; this is true both because the air we breathe is more often contaminated by tubercle bacilli than the food we eat, and also because the mucous membrane of the intestinal tract is more resistant to this type of infection than is the mucous membrane of the respiratory tract. Even rarer are primary infections established by implantation of bacilli through the skin and mucous membranes. Thus, the subcutaneous tissues and the vaginal mucous membrane are sometimes found to be the sites of primary infection.

By whatever route tubercle bacilli penetrate the previously uninfected body, they proceed to multiply locally, causing first acute inflammation and then tubercle formation. In a primary infection, the invading bacilli are not confined to the primary focus, but some of them find their way into the lymphatics and then into the regional lymph nodes (1, 2). From the apex of the lungs tubercle bacilli normally drain to the paratracheal nodes, from the remainder of the lungs they drain to the hilar nodes, and from the intestinal tract to the mesenteric nodes. The primary parenchymal focus and the regional nodes together comprise what is called the primary complex.

The primary parenchymal focus begins as a small area of acute inflammation containing tubercle bacilli. At this stage these bacilli multiply freely and the area of inflammation grows larger, but at first no capsule forms. After a few weeks, tuberculin hypersensitivity develops and the character of the primary focus begins to change. Perifocal infiltration develops, the focus caseates, and the regional nodes enlarge. The enlargement of both the primary focus and the regional nodes may be rapid and great. The size of the primary complex varies with the number of infecting tubercle bacilli and the age and resistance of the patient. Once the acute phase of the primary focus is reached, the lesion usually regresses slowly, over a period of months or even years. The caseous material becomes calcified, and though viable tubercle bacilli may persist for a number of years, eventually the primary focus becomes sterile (3). Drug therapy often results in more rapid and more complete clearing of the primary focus.

Usually the primary focus is benign, but not always. Rarely, the primary lesion progresses even after hypersensitivity develops, and its caseous center liquefies instead of becoming inspissated and calcified. When this happens a tuberculous cavity is formed, and there is a strong tendency for the disease to spread through the bronchi to other parts of the lungs. This progression of the primary lesion is commonest in young infants, and may be serious or even fatal.

Like the primary parenchymal focus, the lymph node component of the primary complex usually regresses spontaneously. However, the enlarged lymph nodes may cause serious damage (1). They may cause obstruction of the bronchi by their size, or the tuberculous infection may progress through the walls of the bronchi, causing tuberculous endobronchitis, swelling of the bronchial mucous membrane, and sometimes bronchial obstruction. If bronchial obstruction occurs and persists for more than a short time, air cannot reach the segment or lobe distal to the point of obstruction, the air already present is absorbed, and that portion of the lung shrinks in size and becomes partly or totally functionless. Usually the shrunken portion of the lung becomes infected and bronchiectatic. Enlarged tuberculous lymph nodes may compress not only the nearby bronchi but other nearby structures as well. Depending on their size and location, these nodes may cause pressure on the esophagus, the blood vessels and the pericardium.

Though the lymph node component of the primary complex is usually benign, this is not always so. The disease process in the nodes may progress locally and cause a fistula into a bronchus, permitting spread of disease by way of the bronchi. Sometimes this process is very dramatic, a large soft caseous node rupturing suddenly into a bronchus and causing acute illness and a massive spread of disease. When tuberculosis is first diagnosed in a child in pneumonic form, the mechanism by which pneumonia was caused may well have been the rupture of such a tuberculous lymph node into the tracheo-bronchial tree.

Immediately after primary infection takes place, the infecting tubercle bacilli are not localized to the area of the primary complex. Tubercle bacilli find their way into the bloodstream, directly or by way of the lymphatics, and are then disseminated throughout the body. This spread by way of the bloodstream takes place at intervals until acquired resistance develops, after which it diminishes and then stops altogether. The foci which develop in various parts of the body in the immediate post-primary period often harbor living tubercle bacilli, and may become the source of later disease. The primary parenchymal focus is seldom the cause of later tuberculous disease, since it usually heals thoroughly and becomes sterile (3); the only important exception is the progressive primary focus with cavity formation, in which tubercle bacilli may persist indefinitely.

The tissue reaction is quite different in primary and in reinfection tuberculosis. In primary infection, as we have seen, the tissue response is relatively slow, the infecting tubercle bacilli are free to find their way into the lymphatics and into the bloodstream, and the regional lymph nodes are involved early and extensively. In reinfection tuberculosis, that is, in infection occurring either from without the body or from the breakdown of a focus within the body after acquired resistance has developed, the inflammatory tissue reaction to the invading bacilli is greatly accelerated. As a result, the bacilli tend to be localized to the site of invasion and are prevented from entering the circulation, and the regional lymph nodes are not involved (4).

The dissemination of tubercle bacilli which occurs during the formation of the primary complex is responsible for most of the tuberculosis which develops later in life. What will happen in an individual case cannot be predicted, because there are so many variables—single or multiple disseminations, number and virulence of the bacilli, natural resistance of the host, and the susceptibility or resistance of the organs or tissues in which the bacilli are deposited (5). Many of the implanted bacilli die, some grow and form tuberculous foci which become quiescent, and some develop into foci of active and progressive tuberculosis. The tuberculous foci which are created in this fashion, whether active or quiescent, may continue to shelter viable bacilli for a very long time, and may evolve into active tuberculosis many years later.

Reinfection tuberculosis may be exogenous or endogenous. The immunity acquired as a result of primary infection protects the individual against most exogenous infections, but the introduction of large numbers of virulent tubercle bacilli can overwhelm this immunity and cause disease (2). Cases have been reported of individuals who had primary infection in the days before antituberculosis chemotherapy was available, who developed typical reinfection pulmonary tuberculosis, whose sputum was positive and whose tubercle bacilli were resistant to streptomycin before chemotherapy was administered. This is strong evidence of exogenous reinfection, since it is highly improbable that in these cases the primary infection was due to streptomycin-resistant tubercle bacilli.

Inoculation tuberculosis is additional evidence of the possibility of exogenous reinfection; a pathologist who inoculates a large number of tubercle bacilli into his fingers by means of a contaminated knife or needle will usually develop a tuberculous nodule at the site of inoculation even though he previously had a primary tuberculous infection. A significant amount of adult pulmonary tuberculosis may be due to exogenous reinfection, but most other forms of tuberculosis in adults and older children are due to the reactivation of tuberculous foci which originated during the dissemination of tubercle bacilli soon after the primary infection occurred. Even adult pulmonary tuberculosis is usually endogenous in origin, arising from tubercle bacilli deposited in the tissues soon after the primary infection.

When tubercle bacilli lodge in the various tissues, there are two ways by which they can cause disease at a later date. In some structures, such as kidneys and bone, the original focus can progress concentrically, causing disease by causing local destruction. In the case of the meninges and the serous cavities, however, a different mechanism is involved.

In miliary tuberculosis, or in experimental tuberculosis in which large numbers of tubercle bacilli are injected into the bloodstream, tubercles develop on the serous surfaces in small numbers, but typical tuberculosis of the meninges, pleura, pericardium, peritoneum or joints, with the production of large amounts of fluid, does not occur. Large numbers of bacilli must be present in the serous cavities of hypersensitive patients or experimental animals in order for tuberculous effusions to take place. This happens when a caseous cerebral tuberculous focus extends and discharges a large number of bacilli into the subarachnoid space, or when an adjacent tuberculous lesion enlarges and heavily infects a serous cavity. Thus, subpleural tubercles or tuberculous lymph nodes may infect the pleura, a tuberculous Fallopian tube may infect the peritoneum, a caseous lymph node may infect the pericardium, and a caseous focus in bone may contaminate a joint. It is worth repeating that the implantation of blood-borne tubercle bacilli on the meninges or serous membranes does not result in disease; disease in these situations is caused by the implantation of tubercle bacilli in adjacent tissues, and then the enlargement of the resulting foci, their caseation, and their rupture, with the discharge of large numbers of tubercle bacilli into the subarachnoid space or into a serous cavity (2).

The pathogenesis of chronic pulmonary tuberculosis is somewhat complicated, and this disease can develop by several mechanisms. The primary parenchymal focus is very seldom the source of reinfection, since in most cases it becomes sterile fairly early. However, tubercle bacilli often persist in the regional lymph nodes for a long time. It is possible for inflammation from these nodes to involve the nearby bronchi, and tubercle bacilli from these nodes may be discharged into the bronchi years later, thus causing chronic pulmonary tuberculosis. In the dissemination of tubercle bacilli which occurs by way of the bloodstream soon after the primary infection, it is common for small tuberculous foci to develop in the apices of the lungs, and later reactivation of these foci may result in chronic pulmonary tuberculosis.

Chronic pulmonary tuberculosis takes many forms, but the commonest involves slowly or intermittently progressive destruction of pulmonary tissue associated with considerable fibrosis. Tubercle bacilli, whether brought to the site through the bronchi or through the bloodstream, usually initiate a caseous focus in the alveoli. Usually the focus heals, but it may grow larger by direct extension or by disseminating bacilli through a small bronchus. Periods of spread of disease alternate with periods of fibrosis. Usually healing occurs without the development of clinical disease, but, since many caseous foci shelter living tubercle bacilli for many years, reactivation and further progression can take place. Ultimately, in those cases in which this process of alternate progression and fibrosis occurs, a considerable local lesion will exist, with cavity formation, repeated dissemination by way of the bronchial tree, and secondary lesions in other parts of the lung (6). The number and virulence of the tubercle bacilli, the degree of hypersensitivity, and the native and acquired resistance of the host will determine whether a given infection will result in a healed scar or in chronic progressive tuberculosis with caseation, fibrosis and cavity formation.

Caseous pneumonia may be due to tubercle bacilli brought to the lungs either by way of the bloodstream or the bronchi. The foci caused by hematogenous dissemination are always small and multiple; they remain small because each focus is due to a small number of bacilli which multiply slowly. The bronchial route is much more commonly involved and is capable of causing areas of caseous pneumonia ranging in size from a few millimeters to an entire lobe. The source of bacilli is softened caseous material. In children, this material may come either from a cavity or from a lymph node which has eroded a bronchus. In adults, extensive caseation of lymph nodes is uncommon, so the bacilli which are responsible for bronchogenic caseous pneumonia are usually aspirated from a tuberculous cavity. It is important to remember that tuberculous pneumonia of considerable extent cannot be due to the rapid spread of tuberculous infection from a few bacilli, since these bacilli multiply slowly. Extensive or lobar tuberculous pneumonia can be caused only by the sudden aspiration of large numbers of tubercle bacilli, from a cavity or softened caseous node, into the entire involved area.

SUMMARY

Tubercle bacilli enter the body, usually by way of the respiratory or alimentary tract, and establish a primary infection. During the next few weeks the bacilli do not remain localized, but make their way into the lymphatics and regional nodes, and in small numbers they are often disseminated throughout the body by way of the bloodstream.

The primary parenchymal focus and the tuberculous regional nodes together constitute the primary complex. A few weeks after the primary infection occurs immunity develops, and thereafter the tubercle bacilli tend to be localized. It is the bacilli which have been disseminated from the primary parenchymal focus which are the cause of much disease later in life.

Uusally the primary parenchymal focus is benign, but sometimes it progresses and forms a cavity. Usually the lymph node component is benign, but these enlarged nodes can cause trouble by mechanical pressure, and they are more likely to caseate and spread disease than the parenchymal focus.

Most of the tubercle bacilli which reach the tissues in the early weeks after primary infection die, but some establish themselves, grow and produce secondary foci of infection. Many of these foci become quiescent, but some progress. In either case, viable bacilli persist in these foci for a long time, and these may produce progressive disease many years later. In organs such as the kidneys, disease may arise directly by progression from such foci. In other structures, such as the meninges or the serous cavities, disease is due to the presence of a caseous focus nearby, which grows and ultimately discharges large numbers of bacilli into the subarachnoid space or the serous cavity.

In the lungs, foci are established after the primary infection, either from an exogenous source or by a spread from an endogenous source by way of the bloodstream or bronchi. Once established, caseation may develop, followed by softening and cavity formation. Alternate periods of bronchial spread followed by healing and fibrosis may result in healing or in chronic pulmonary tuberculosis. Factors which influence the outcome are the number and virulence of the bacilli, the degree of hypersensitivity, and the native and acquired resistance of the host.

REFERENCES

1. LINCOLN, E. M., AND SEWELL, E. M.: *Tuberculosis in Children*. New York, McGraw-Hill, 1963.
2. RICH, A. R.: *The Pathogenesis of Tuberculosis*, 2nd ed., Springfield, Thomas, 1951.
3. FELDMAN, W. H., AND BAGGENSTOSS, A. H.: The residual infectivity

of the primary complex of tuberculosis. *Amer. J. Path., 14*:473, 1938.

4. LINCOLN, E. M., GILBERT, L., AND MORALES, S. M.: Chronic pulmonary tuberculosis in individuals with known previous primary tuberculosis, *Dis. Chest, 38*:473, 1960.

5. LURIE, M. B., ZAPPASODI, P., AND TICKNER, C.: On the nature of genetic resistance to tuberculosis in the light of the host-parasite relationship in natively resistant and susceptible rabbits. *Amer. Rev. Tuberc., 72*:297, 1955.

6. MEDLAR, E. M.: The behavior of pulmonary tuberculous lesions: A pathological study. *Amer. Rev. Tuberc., 71*: March, Part 2, 1955.

Chapter III

BASIC PRINCIPLES OF DRUG TREATMENT IN TUBERCULOSIS

By DRUG TREATMENT, we mean treatment with drugs which have an inhibitory effect on tubercle bacilli in the human body. Drugs which are effective in the test tube but not in the body are excluded from discussion. Excluded also are drugs which offer symptomatic benefit only.

Development of clinical tuberculosis requires not only infection with tubercle bacilli but also the growth and multiplication of the bacteria until they are numerous enough to cause significant tissue damage. A drug is effective in the treatment of tuberculosis if it is capable of killing the bacilli, or if it is capable of interfering with their growth and multiplication and thereby preventing an increase in their number. As none of our antituberculosis drugs are actually bactericidal in the doses used, the normal body defenses must be relied upon to fix, and eventually to destroy, the organisms present at the time drug treatment is started. In most cases these body defenses are entirely adequate, once the multiplication of organisms has been stopped.

When a drug is evaluated to decide whether it will be effective, information is needed as to its effectiveness and toxicity and the rapidity with which bacilli develop resistance to it.

The effectiveness of a drug depends in part on its ability to reach the bacilli in concentrations great enough to inhibit their growth or multiplication. If it is given by mouth, the drug must be well absorbed from the gastrointestinal tract. By whatever route it is given, the drug must reach the tuberculous lesion in a good concentration. Since the principal mode by which drugs reach the lesion is by way of the bloodstream, the availability of a good blood supply in the region of the lesion is very helpful. This is the reason why good drugs produce their most dramatic results in fresh exudative lesions; these

[16]

lesions are associated with hyperemia, and because of this they regularly show a higher concentration of the drugs than does normal tissue. Scarred lesions are relatively avascular, so the amount of drugs in these lesions is reduced. This is not important, though, since scarred lesions contain few bacilli. Necrotic lesions have no blood supply. To be effective in necrotic lesions, the drug must therefore be capable of penetrating them by diffusion. This is extremely important, since, as Canetti has well shown, softened necrotic foci contain very numerous bacilli. Most important of all, an effective drug must be able to penetrate the walls of tuberculous cavities and to inhibit the growth of bacilli there. The cavity is, of all tuberculous lesions, the most fraught with danger. This is true because conditions in the cavity wall favor the growth and multiplication of tubercle bacilli, and because the open bronchi favor the spread of these bacilli throughout the lungs. Even microscopic cavities are dangerous. So long as bacilli persist in the walls of cavities the patient is in danger of relapse.

Of course a drug needs to have other qualities than the ability to reach the bacilli in high concentration, in order to be an effective antituberculosis drug. It must be toxic for tubercle bacilli and either nontoxic or of low toxicity for human beings. The mechanism of action on the bacilli may vary, but somehow the effective drug must interfere with the essential life processes, or the growth or multiplication of the bacilli. There are many possible modes of action by which a drug may accomplish this. It may inhibit the uptake of essential cellular constituents; it may block the synthesis of products essential for cellular welfare; it may prevent the excretion of cellular waste products, or it may act in many other manners. The effect of its contact with bacterial cells may be so damaging that the cells die, and in this case the drug has a bactericidal effect. This state of affairs does not occur with any of the antituberculosis drugs in the doses in which they are used in man or experimental animals, but it does occur in some cases in the test tube, when very high concentrations of the drug can be obtained and the pH can be manipulated. Commonly, the effect of the use of drugs on tubercle bacilli is to inhibit the process of cell division by interfering with the action of an enzyme system necessary for cell division, such as the oxidation-reduction reaction.

This does not destroy the bacilli, but effectively prevents their multiplication.

Toxicity of the drug for body cells is one of the factors which limits the usefulness of antituberculosis drugs or in some cases prevents their use altogether. Potent drugs are likely to have more than one action, and though their adverse effect on tubercle bacilli is desirable, some of their other actions may be undesirable or even dangerous. Some toxic manifestations are merely unpleasant, and may be accepted as a price that must be paid for the use of a useful drug. Others, however, may cause real injury to the patient or even threaten his life, and in these cases, of course, the drug must be discontinued at once. If serious toxicity from a drug is common, that drug may have little or no usefulness, no matter how effective it is in the test tube or in experimental animals.

The toxic manifestations of drugs useful in the treatment of tuberculosis cover a wide range, including damage to brain, cranial nerves and peripheral nerves, injury to liver and kidneys and blood-forming organs, irritation of the gastrointestinal tract and many, many more. The specific toxicity which may occur from each drug will be discussed as the value and usefulness of each drug is discussed. It is important to be aware of the toxicity of each drug, so that treatment may be planned intelligently. Clearly, needless risk is involved in giving a hepatotoxic drug to patients who already have damaged livers, or in giving a psychotoxic drug to a patient with a history of psychosis. Even when the drugs have been selected wisely, it is important to recognize their potential toxicity, so that the proper examinations can be made and treatment changed early if evidence of toxicity develops.

In addition to strictly toxic manifestations, some drugs may cause allergic reactions in susceptible individuals. These reactions are not related to the drug's pharmacologic action, and are not related to dose or cumulative action. For instance, in certain individuals, doses of streptomycin too small to have any clinical effect may cause very severe allergic reactions. There is no way of predicting what patients will have allergic reactions to particular drugs, but patients who have a history of other allergic manifestations are much more likely to have drug allergies than are patients with no such history. Also, patients with severe, acute infections such as lobar pneumonia are more likely to have allergic drug reactions than patients with chronic infections. The manifestations of drug allergies run the full gamut of hypersensitivity reactions. The most common manifestations of allergic drug reactions may be divided into hematological, dermatological, neurological, gastrointestinal and miscellaneous. The most common hematological reactions are leukocytosis, lymphocytosis, anemia and eosinophilia. The most common skin reactions are morbilliform, maculopapular and urticarial, but vesicular, purpuric and even exfoliative lesions are also seen and pruritus is common. Among neurological reactions, delirium, peripheral neuritis and anesthesias and paresthesias are the most frequent. Nausea, vomiting, diarrhoea and abdominal pain are the most common gastrointestinal reactions. Drug fever may occur alone or with other manifestations of drug allergy. It is often accompanied by chills, constitutional symptoms and leukocytosis, and usually appears abruptly, though sometimes the temperature rises to a maximum in a series of steps. Jaundice is a response which may be due to a variety of agents. Renal disorders, periarteritis nodosa and systemic lupus erythematosus are formidable, but fortunately uncommon, drug reactions.

Allergic drug reactions usually require only the prompt withdrawal of the offending drug. When this is done, the reactions usually come to an end promptly. Sometimes, however, the reactions persist or recur; thus, exfoliative dermatitis may persist for a long time after the causative drug has been discontinued, and urticaria may recur for weeks or months even though the drug which caused it is no longer used. When drug allergy is severe or persistent, adrenocortical steroids are usually indicated, though antihistamines or epinephrine may be enough to control the situation.

When a patient has had an allergic reaction to an antituberculosis drug, that drug should ordinarily never be used again, because even the administration of a single small dose is likely to precipitate a new reaction. Occasionally no other drug is available, so that it is necessary to use the same drug again. When this happens, the simultaneous use of adrenocortical steroids usually suppresses the allergic manifestations.

One of the phenomena that limits the usefulness of good drugs is the development by the bacteria of resistance to those drugs. When resistance develops, the bacteria are able to grow and multiply again in the presence of the drugs, which have lost the ability to inhibit them. Since the treatment of tuberculosis requires two years or thereabouts, the development of drug resistance in a shorter period of time may be a serious matter.

It was formerly thought that drug-resistant bacteria developed gradually by physiologic adaption to the drugs to which they were exposed. This view is no longer widely held. Any population of tubercle bacilli is not entirely homogeneous. Spontaneous mutations occur, so that at any time there are a small number of mutants in the population. These mutants are no better equipped to survive and grow than their normal counterparts, so under ordinary conditions they remain few and unimportant. The mutation rate for streptomycin-resistant bacilli is about one per million, and these resistant bacilli grow no more rapidly, nor are they more virulent, than the normal bacilli from which they arose, so under normal circumstances they pass unnoticed. When streptomycin is given to such a bacterial population, the 999,999 susceptible organisms are inhibited from multiplying, but the one resistant cell in a million can grow and multiply freely, so that in a few months all the bacilli present in the lesions are resistant to streptomycin. Streptomycin does not cause the resistant mutants to develop, but by inhibiting the growth of the susceptible bacilli it eventually permits the descendants of the resistant bacilli to become dominant in the bacterial population. This is known as "selection under pressure."

When streptomycin was the only available antituberculosis drug, this meant that drug treatment offered only a temporary check to the growth of bacilli. A period of three or four months existed, during which the patient often felt better and during which the progress of disease was halted. During this short period, resectional surgery might be carried out with a measure of safety, or the patient's own resistance might suffice to heal the disease. However, usually after this short respite of three or four months, laboratory examinations would show that the tubercle bacilli had become streptomycin resistant and the disease again began to progress. However, when two effective drugs became available, the situation changed markedly. If mutants resistant to streptomycin arise with a frequency of one in a million, and if mutants resistant to a second drug arise with the same frequency, a mutant resistant to both drugs could be expected to occur with a frequency of one in 1,000,000 x 1,000,000, or one in a trillion. If two effective drugs are used simultaneously, the bacteria in the lesion are usually suppressed entirely and the sputum becomes negative. The conversion of sputum to negative is a vital step in the treatment of tuberculosis, since it minimizes both the risk of relapse for the patient and the risk of transmitting the infection to others.

Since a number of effective drugs now exist, it is almost always possible to choose a combination which will inhibit the bacilli and permit the body to heal the disease. The first drugs to be considered are the three basic drugs, isoniazid, streptomycin and paraminosalicylic acid (PAS), and a combination of any two of these drugs is usually perfectly adequate. If, however, some of these drugs cannot be used, because of toxicity, or hypersensitivity, or if they are unlikely to be effective because resistance exists, we can choose from among a considerable array of second-line drugs. These include viomycin, cycloserine, pyrazinamide, ethionamide, kanamycin, and others. These are usually kept in reserve, because they are more toxic, more expensive and less effective than the basic drugs, but when needed they frequently can do the job.

Treatment failure is usually due to inadequate treatment. Inadequate treatment means interrupted treatment, a too-brief course of treatment, or treatment with the wrong drugs. Interruption of treatment has many causes, but the commonest cause is the failure of the patient to understand the need for long, tedious months of taking drugs when he feels good and has been informed that his sputum is negative and his x-rays are satisfactory. Interruption of treatment sometimes leads to relapse, and too often leads to the development of resistant bacilli. A too-brief course of treatment is usually any period of treatment lasting less than two years. Since the duration of hospitalization is generally only a few months, why must drugs be given for two years? The practical reason is that shorter periods of treatment are often proved to be insufficient because a significant percentage of them are followed by relapses. This is easily explained because, effective as the drugs are, they usually act only on the bacterial cells which are ready to divide, so that resting cells are not affected. It is therefore desirable to continue giving drugs for a long time, so as to interfere with the process of cell division in as many bacilli as possible. Treatment with the wrong drugs has also been mentioned above as a cause of treatment failure. There are, of course, intrinsically no "wrong drugs." Yet in the management of an individual patient, persisting in the use of a given drug combination after the patient's disease has begun to show progression, or after the laboratory tests have shown drug resistance, is risky. In this situation the "wrong drugs" are probably being used. The therapy should be reevaluated, and in most cases the drugs should be changed.

SUMMARY

The value of a drug in the treatment of tuberculosis depends on its effectiveness, toxicity, and the rapidity with which tubercle bacilli become resistant to it. Its effectiveness depends on its ability to inhibit vital life processes of tubercle bacilli or their capability for growth or multiplication. Its toxicity means its adverse effect on the cells of the patient, and in an ideal drug this should be minimal; serious toxicity severely limits the usefulness of even a very good drug. Resistance is an unfortunate property of bacteria whereby, following exposure to a drug, they acquire the ability to live, grow and multiply in its presence. Resistance to a drug can be postponed by using drugs in pairs rather than singly. The initial course of treatment offers the best opportunity for healing the tuberculous lesion. The commonest cause of treatment failure is inadequate treatment—interrupted treatment, too short a course of treatment, or treatment with ineffective drugs, or drugs in an ineffective dosage.

Chapter IV

THE BASIC DRUGS

It is not entirely logical to divide the antituberculosis drugs into two groups, "basic" and "secondary." Such a division implies that the "secondary" drugs are inferior, and although this may be true in some cases, it is by no means true in all cases. When treating an individual patient, the selection of drugs should be made on the basis of his history of previous drug treatment and of the laboratory reports of bacterial susceptibility to the various drugs. For instance, if a patient gives a history of six months' treatment with isoniazid and PAS, and if the laboratory reports that his tubercle bacilli are resistant to these two drugs, his treatment should be based on two other drugs. Drugs which inhibit the tubercle bacilli should always be used; whether they are "basic" or "secondary" is of little importance.

Nevertheless, there are reasons why it is useful to consider the antituberculosis drugs in these two groups. The "basic" or "primary" drugs—isoniazid, streptomycin and PAS—have been available longer than the others, so that we are most familiar with them. Two drug combinations selected from this group of three are usually highly effective in the treatment of patients who have not received these drugs before, and these two-drug combinations seldom produce serious toxicity. These drugs are also relatively inexpensive, and because of this and their freedom from serious toxicity, they are usually available from out-patient clinics for the treatment of patients at home. The situation is quite different with the "secondary" drugs. Generally more toxic, less effective, and more expensive than the "basic" drugs, they require much more supervision, and as a result they are usually reserved for patients receiving treatment in hospitals. In this chapter the three basic drugs will be considered.

ISONIAZID

Isoniazid (isonicotinic acid hydrazide) is the most valuable of the antituberculosis drugs. It has all the virtues of a good drug — it is highly effective; it is readily absorbed from the gastrointestinal tract; it is widely distributed throughout the body; it not only diffuses into caseous masses but is concentrated in them; it is of low toxicity, and it is inexpensive.

Isoniazid was synthesized in 1912, and its chemical properties were explored at that time, but its value as a drug was unsuspected for almost forty years. It was not until the possible antituberculosis value of the thiosemicarbazones came to be investigated that isoniazid was noticed, and then only by chance, because it was used as one step in a chemical process leading to the synthesis of a derivative of the thiosemicarbazone of isonicotinylaldehyde. The thiosemicarbazone proved only slightly active, but, about 1950, several drug companies began investigating the value of this intermediary, isoniazid, in tuberculosis, and the first report of its great value was made in 1952 (1).

Isoniazid is a white or colorless crystalline powder, odorless, and freely soluble in water. For adults the average dose is about 5 mg per kg, while children may receive a daily dose of 5 mg to 10 mg per kg. The average oral daily dose for adults is therefore about 300 mg, which may be given in a single dose or in divided doses; the most frequently used regimen is 100 mg three times daily. There are preparations available for parenteral use, but there is little need for them since the oral drug is so rapidly absorbed and so widely distributed.

Following oral administration, isoniazid is rapidly absorbed. A single oral dose of 3 mg per kg results in blood concentrations of 1.3 to 3.4 μg per ml in about an hour (2). The blood level gradually decreases to 0.2 μg per ml in six hours, and low but detectable levels may persist as long as twenty-four hours. Parenteral administration produces higher peaks but less prolonged levels. The use of C^{14}-labelled isoniazid (3) has given us a great deal of information concerning the distribution of the drug in the tissues. The drug appears in kidneys, spleen, muscle, lungs, brain, intestines, liver and skin. It appears in saliva, pleural fluid, cerebrospinal fluid and milk. It passes the placental barrier freely, and is present in the fetal blood and tissues (4). Isoniazid penetrates the capsule of tubercles and diffuses into their necrotic centers. There is selective accumulation of the drug in certain tissues. Twenty-four hours after its administration, the liver, skin, lungs and caseous material still retain considerable amounts, while the drug has disappeared from other tissues such as brain and muscle. Four days after the last oral dose, tuberculostatic concentrations of isoniazid are still to be found in caseous masses. Administration of isoniazid several times daily instead of once daily further increases the selective concentration of the drug, especially in caseous tissue. The distribution of isoniazid is not affected by the simultaneous administration of PAS. The concentration of the drug in the normal cerebrospinal fluid is ordinarily about one-fifth of the plasma concentration, but in patients with tuberculous meningitis much higher concentrations are reached. Apparently the permeability of the meninges is increased by inflammation, so that after a dose of 3 mg per kg is administered to a patient with tuberculous meningitis, a drug concentration of 4 μg per ml is often achieved in the cerebrospinal fluid. This is high enough to be tuberculostatic. Excretion studies have shown that 75 to 95 per cent of ingested isoniazid is excreted in the urine in the first twenty-four hours. Less than 1 per cent is excreted in the feces, and almost none is excreted in the breath. Neither pyridoxine nor PAS influence plasma levels nor the rate of urinary excretion. On prolonged administration, there is no accumulation of the drug in blood or tissues.

After isoniazid is absorbed, some of it remains in the form of free isoniazid, and some is conjugated to acetyl isoniazid. Smaller amounts are changed in the body to isonicotinoyl hydrazone, N-methyl isoniazid, and isonicotinyl glycine. Of all these, only free isoniazid is an effective tuberculostatic agent; all the other forms are inactive, or almost inactive, against tubercle bacilli. The ability to conjugate isoniazid to less effective drugs varies widely in different people. For a time it was hoped that the "rapid inactivators" of isoniazid could be treated just as effectively as the "slow inactivators," compensating for the isoniazid which was lost through acetylation by giving larger doses of the drug. It now appears that increasing the dose is not helpful in this situation; those who acetylate and inactivate isoniazid rapidly do not respond quite as well to isoniazid regardless of dose, but they usually make an adequate response.

Though the ability to acetylate isoniazid varies greatly in different people, it is constant throughout life in the same individual.

Isoniazid is a highly specific drug, being active against human and bovine strains of tubercle bacilli and against no other bacteria. Isoniazid is an antimetabolite. High concentrations inhibit endogenous respiration of tubercle bacilli. Isoniazid also inhibits the oxidation of pyruvate, lactate, acetate, glucose and glycerol (5). Isoniazid does not act on resting tubercle bacilli, but, whatever its mode of action, it is effective only against actively growing and multiplying tubercle bacilli. So active is isoniazid that susceptible bacilli are inhibited in the test tube by concentrations as low as 0.05 μg per ml. Since plasma concentrations more than twenty times higher than this can readily be obtained by oral dosage, and since isoniazid accumulates selectively in areas of active tuberculous inflammation, it can be seen that isoniazid given orally is a highly effective drug. This wide margin, between the inhibitory level and the level actually achieved in the plasma by average oral doses, also explains why isoniazid is effective even in the case of the rapid inactivators of the drug, because even though half or more of the drug is inactivated, the remainder is still greater than the small amount needed for inhibition. When isoniazid was originally used alone in the treatment of tuberculosis, it proved to be extremely effective. Symptomatic treatment was prompt and great — temperature subsided, cough decreased, sputum volume diminished, appetite improved and weight increased. So dramatic was the clinical improvement and the consequent feeling of well-being, that the patients were described as "dancing in the aisles" of their hospital wards. Pulmonary lesions showed improvement by x-ray in a short time; sputum sometimes became negative in a few weeks, and lesions of the mouth, tongue, intestinal tract, larynx, bronchi and kidneys responded promptly (1). Even in miliary and meningeal tuberculosis, isoniazid proved to be a highly effective drug. Isoniazid is not only widely distributed in the intercellular spaces but penetrates the cells themselves, and is just as effective against intracellular as against extracellular tubercle bacilli.

These excellent results were obtained by using isoniazid alone. It is rarely desirable to use this drug alone in the treatment of active tuberculosis because resistance develops rapidly, and this somewhat limits its effectiveness. It will be seen later that isoniazid-resistance may not have the same significance as streptomycin-resistance, but it is undesirable just the same. Used in conjunction with an effective companion drug such as PAS or streptomycin, the therapeutic effect of the combined drugs is a little greater in the first month or two and is far more long-lasting, and in a high percentage of cases results in a clinical cure.

The clinical toxicity of isoniazid is relatively slight. The commonest toxic manifestation is peripheral neuritis, which occurs infrequently when the standard dose of 5 mg per kg is used. With larger doses, anesthesia, paresthesia, burning and pain along the distribution of sensory nerves in the extremities is not uncommon, occurring in ten to fifteen per cent of patients who take 10 mg per kg or more (6). It has been found that isoniazid depletes the tissues of pyridoxine by the formation and excretion of isonicotinyl hydrazone of pyridoxal (7) in the urine, and that this peripheral neuritis can be prevented by the administration of pyridoxine in doses of 50 mg once or twice daily. It has also been shown that pyridoxine does not reduce the therapeutic effectiveness of isoniazid. In children, pyridoxine deficiency almost never occurs during isoniazid therapy, and in young adults it is less frequent and less severe than in older persons. When using isoniazid in doses of more than 5 mg per kg in adults it is therefore a good plan to administer pyridoxine concurrently; when isoniazid is used in doses of 5 mg per kg or less, the administration of pyridoxine is not necessary.

Large doses of isoniazid have been reported to cause central nervous system stimulation, with restlessness, loss of ability to concentrate, insomnia, muscle twitching and increased reflexes. These symptoms are seldom severe and are usually transient, disappearing during the course of continued administration of the drug. Very large doses, 40 mg per kg or higher, have been known to cause convulsions, but these doses are far above the therapeutic range and need never be used in the treatment of tuberculosis. It is perfectly safe to give isoniazid in doses of 5 mg per kg to epileptic patients who are receiving anticonvulsant therapy; such patients are no more likely to develop convulsions than if they were not receiving isoniazid.

It has been said that patients receiving isoniazid sometimes develop psychoses, but investigations show that this is quite rare, and it is doubtful that the drug was causally related to the psychosis. It is safe to give isoniazid to psychotic patients without danger of causing an exacerbation, and it is safe to give isoniazid to nonpsychotic patients without risk of precipitating a psychosis.

Hypersensitivity reactions occur in about 1 per cent of patients who receive isoniazid. These reactions take the form of drug fever, rashes and hepatitis; these manifestations may occur singly or in combination. If isoniazid is being given with PAS, and a hypersensitivity reaction to PAS occurs, cross-hypersensitivity to isoniazid is likely to develop. Almost all patients who are hypersensitive to isoniazid can be desensitized, using very small and gradually increasing doses of the drug by mouth. The following schedule will produce desensitization in most cases.

ORAL INH DESENSITIZATION

Days	Dose of INH in Milligrams	Number of Doses Daily
1	0.01	1
2	0.02	1
3	0.05	1
4	0.1	1
5	0.2	1
6	0.5	1
7	1.0	1
8	2.0	1
9	4.0	1
.	.	.
.	.	.
.	.	.
.	(Dose of INH Increased by 2 mg Daily)	.
.	.	.
.	.	.
.	.	.
41	68	1
42	70	1
43	75	1
44	80	1
45	85	1
46	90	1
47	95	1
48	100	1
49	100	2
50	100	3

Rapid desensitization can also be carried out, using steroids along with increasing doses of isoniazid. On four successive days the patient may receive prednisone or another adrenocorticosteroid hormone, accompanied by isoniazid in doses of 25 mg three times daily, the first day; 50 mg three times daily, the second; 75 mg three times daily, the third day, and 100 mg three times daily on the fourth day. Then the steroid is tapered off and the isoniazid is continued.

When isoniazid was first used, there were already a few strains of tubercle bacilli which exhibited varying degrees of resistance to it; occasionally this initial resistance was significant, but most frequently it was of a lower order and did not interfere with treatment. Now, more than ten years later, the incidence of significant primary drug resistance is still low, being perhaps 4 or 5 per cent (8). The increase is probably due to infection with tubercle bacilli derived from patients who have received unsuccesful treatment.

Following treatment with isoniazid alone, drug resistance appears in a short time, usually a few weeks; in some cases resistance may be delayed for as long as twenty-eight weeks even when the drug is used alone. When isoniazid is used with another effective drug, the sputum usually becomes negative in a few months. However, when the sputum remains positive, the tubercle bacilli finally become resistant to both drugs.

The clinical significance of *in vitro* resistance to isoniazid is hard to determine. In the case of streptomycin, the development of resistance in the test tube spells the end of the usefulness of that drug in treatment of a patient harboring that strain of bacilli; resistance in the test tube means that the value of that drug has been lost in that particular patient. The same thing seems to be true with most of the other antituberculosis drugs; *in vitro* resistance and *in vivo* resistance are about the same. In the case of isoniazid this principle often does not apply. Tubercle bacilli may not be inhibited by isoniazid in the test tube and yet the drug may continue to be effective therapeutically. This was well shown in the autopsy material in the early days of isoniazid therapy. Patients whose chemotherapy was stopped because of the development of resistance to isoniazid frequently died with extensive tuberculous ulceration of the intestinal tract. Similar patients also harboring isoniazid resistant tubercle bacilli, who continued to take isoniazid, sometimes recovered and sometimes transformed their pulmonary disease to a much less progressive form; even those who finally succumbed had few or no tuberculous ulcers in the intestinal tract. The exact meaning of *in vitro* resistance to isoniazid is not entirely understood, but it does not have the same unfavorable meaning as does resistance to streptomycin.

Isoniazid-resistant tubercle bacilli frequently have, or develop, a deficiency in catalase activity and many strains of tubercle bacilli with no catalase activity are of reduced virulence. Some of these organisms fail to cause progressive disease in man or monkeys. It is not safe to assume, however, that all isoniazid-resistant catalase-negative tubercle bacilli are without virulence. Patients have been discovered who have never been treated but whose lesions contain only isoniazid-resistant, catalase-negative tubercle bacilli. It must be assumed that these patients were infected with these organisms, which were capable of implanting themselves, multiplying and causing clinical disease. Some patients have died of progressive tuberculosis and only catalase-negative organisms were found in their lesions. Florid, rapidly-progressive disease is seldom caused by catalase-negative bacilli, but some of them, at least, retain enough virulence to cause progressive disease in the patients who harbor them, and to infect and cause clinical disease in other human beings.

Summary

Isoniazid is an extremely useful drug. It is fully effective when administered by mouth. It is rapidly absorbed from the gastro-intestinal tract, is widely distributed throughout the body, and is concentrated and retained in caseous masses. It is active against growing and multiplying tubercle bacilli rather than against resting bacilli. Its dose for adults is 300 mg daily, which may be administered as a single dose or as divided doses; the most widely used dosage schedule is 100 mg three times daily. It is best used in combination with another effective drug, usually streptomycin or PAS. Its toxicity is slight, the most common being peripheral neuritis. This can usually be prevented by the simultaneous use of pyridoxine (50 mg once or twice daily) when isoniazid is used in doses greater than 300 mg daily. Hypersensitivity to isoniazid is uncommon, and most patients who become hypersensitive can be desensitized. The development of resistance is less of a problem than is the case with most other drugs, since clinical refractoriness often does not accompany laboratory evidence of isoniazid resistance.

Isoniazid is our very best antituberculosis drug — the most effective and the least toxic of all the drugs in our armamentarium.

STREPTOMYCIN

Streptomycin was discovered by Waksman and his colleagues in 1944 (9). For many years Professor Waksman had been working on the characteristics of soil microorganisms, especially actinomycetes, believing that many of them exert an antagonistic influence on other organisms. This was not a new idea. It was known as long ago as 1890 that certain of the actinomycetes have the ability to destroy bacteria and fungi, and in the 1920's it was found that this antibacterial activity was selective, a specific actinomycete being active against one or more specific bacteria. Waksman engaged in a systematic study of soil specimens, and showed that a high percentage of the actinomycetes isolated from them had a significant antagonism to fungi, gram-positive bacteria and viruses. Until 1939 all this work was done with living organisms, but at that time a series of antibiotics was prepared from various actinomycetes, and the study progressed using these purified antibiotics. Many of these antibiotics, like the actinomyces which produce them, were shown to be effective against fungi, bacteria and viruses. Some of the antibiotics discovered in these early studies were not effective against disease-producing micoorganisms and some were too toxic for use in animals or man. The first valuable antibiotic to be isolated from an actinomycete was streptomycin. This was derived from an organism called Streptomyces Griseus, and was found to be effective against a variety of bacteria and especially against tubercle bacilli. The finding of streptomycin was the climax of a carefully planned and long-continued search for antibiotics among soil microorganisms, and is one of the success stories of medical research.

Streptomycin has been given in the form of the hydrochloride, the calcium chloride complex, the phosphate, the pantothenate and the sulfate. By far the most commonly used salt is the sulfate. Streptomycin itself is a base, but in this form it is not available.

Streptomycin is a white powder, hygroscopic and freely soluble in water. The streptomycin molecule is composed of streptidine and streptobiosamine, linked together by a glycoside linkage. Streptomycin and its salts are stable at room temperature, retaining their full potency for several years. At higher temperatures deterioration is more rapid. Exposure to light and air do not cause deterioration, but exposure to moisture results in rapid absorption of water. Aqueous solutions of streptomycin darken on exposure to light, but this does not result in loss of potency. Solutions of streptomycin in the p^H range of 3 to 7 are stable for a week or longer at room temperature, and for three months or longer when kept in the refrigerator. Solutions prepared with preservatives retain their potency for prolonged periods at room temperature.

Streptomycin is absorbed poorly, if at all, from the gut. When streptomycin is given by mouth, there are no detectable blood levels, and the drug can be recovered unchanged from the feces to the extent of almost 100 per cent. The oral route of administration may be desirable in some circumstances (for instance, in preparation for surgery of the gastrointestinal tract), but it has no value in the treatment of tuberculosis, for here a systemic effect is required. When the drug is given intramuscularly, absorption is rapid and peak levels are present in the blood stream in one to two hours. The drug disappears from the blood stream more slowly than penicillin; effective blood levels are maintained for about twelve hours, and detectable amounts are still present in twenty-four hours. Streptomycin diffuses into pleural, pericardial, peritoneal and synovial fluids. It does not pass readily through the normal meninges, but, when meningitis is present, the drug appears in the cerebrospinal fluid. It diffuses rapidly through the placenta, and appears in the amniotic fluid and fetal circulation within a few minutes after injection into the mother; the concentration in fetal blood seldom exceeds half the concentration in the mother's blood. The antibiotic appears in saliva, in the bile and in the milk. In the tissues streptomycin appears primarily in the extracellular fluid, as it seems not to penetrate well into the cells themselves (10). It does not penetrate large caseous masses well.

The major excretory pathway is by way of the urinary tract. Streptomycin is excreted by renal glomerular filtration; there is no evidence of either excretion or reabsorption by the tubules. The rate of urinary excretion is most rapid when the blood levels are highest, and most of the drug is excreted unchanged in twenty-four hours. Minor routes of excretion are the biliary pathway, the bowel and the perspiration. Repeated injections do not produce any accumulation of the drug unless there is kidney damage.

Streptomycin is most effective when given intramuscularly in doses of 1 gm daily. In this dosage, toxic manifestations are fairly common, so in many cases it is desirable to reduce the dose either to 0.5 gm daily or to 1 gm twice weekly. These reduced doses are almost, but not quite, as effective as the larger dose. If there is preexisting damage to kidney function, the smaller doses should always be given, since there is likely to be retention of the drug, with higher blood and tissue levels. Oral use of streptomycin is ineffective in tuberculosis, since the drug is not absorbed from the gastrointestinal tract. Subcutaneous injection causes severe local irritation and offers no advantage, so this route of administration is not recommended.

Antituberculosis drugs are rarely used alone, but since streptomycin was the first highly effective antituberculosis drug to be discovered, a great deal of information became available as to its value before combined therapy was introduced. Proof of its effectiveness was firmly established when patients with tuberculous meningitis, treated with streptomycin alone, survived; previously there had been no satisfactory treatment for this disease, which was always fatal. The prolongation of life, and sometimes even the survival, of patients with tuberculous meningitis proved conclusively that streptomycin was an extremely valuable antituberculosis drug (11). The drug was likewise found to be of value in all other kinds of tuberculosis. In pulmonary tuberculosis, clearing of exudative disease was the rule and conversion of sputum was common. Tuberculous lesions of the mucous membranes healed as if by magic, buccal, laryngeal, tracheobronchial and intestinal ulcers healing in a few weeks. The ulcers of the larynx, which had made swallowing and even breathing painful, and the intestinal ulcers, which made life a hell by the violence of the cramps and diarrhoea they caused, were no longer to be feared. Draining tuberculous sinuses and fistulas also healed well, though not quite as rapidly as mucous membrane lesions.

Indeed, one may call the roll of all forms of tuberculosis — genitourinary tuberculosis, tuberculosis of the bones and joints, lymphadenitis, tuberculosis of the eye, ear, skin, pericardium, pleura and other structures — streptomycin is useful in all of them. Streptomycin has proved helpful in the treatment of tuberculosis of every organ and structure in the body (12). It seemed as though this drug by itself, might be able to cure tuberculosis. Two things prevented this from coming to pass — the development of resistance to streptomycin on the part of tubercle bacilli, and the toxicity of the drug.

The excellent initial results of streptomycin treatment are not always maintained. Sinuses, fistulas, and disease of the mucous membranes may heal thoroughly in a few weeks, and may remain healed, without relapsing, even after treatment is stopped. However, most forms of tuberculosis require a much longer period of treatment before cure takes place. Pleural, pulmonary, renal and skeletal tuberculosis for instance, should be treated with effective drugs for two years or longer.

When streptomycin was used alone in these chronic forms of tuberculosis, the initial response was extremely good. In pulmonary tuberculosis, for instance, there was usually reduction in fever, improvement in appetite, gain in weight, reduction in sputum volume, dramatic clearing of exudative lesions, and frequently conversion of sputum. This improvement continued for two or three months, or rarely for four months, and then not only did further improvement cease, but often the disease began to progress again. The tubercle bacilli had become resistant, or rather the resistant strains had multiplied while the susceptible strains had been inhibited, so that the bacillary population which existed after a few months of treatment with streptomycin was no longer inhibited by this drug.

It was shown early that about 75 per cent of all patients who receive streptomycin daily for four months without a companion drug develop resistant tubercle bacilli. Once this happens the drug is no longer helpful in the treatment of the disease. Streptomycin-resistant bacilli are as virulent as susceptible bacilli, so when the bacillary population has become resistant, progression of disease can occur even though streptomycin continues to be given. Such progression was common when streptomycin was given alone, several months of improvement being followed by clinical, bacteriological and radiological relapse.

In the days when streptomycin therapy was the only available form of chemotherapy, it was of the greatest importance to coordinate surgery and drug therapy, timing the thoracic operation (when it was desirable and feasible) so that it was performed after the patient had received considerable benefit from the drug but before the bacilli had become drug-resistant. Streptomycin resistance is a very serious occurrence, because it brings to an end the usefulness of the drug in the patient who has developed resistant organisms; the phenomenon of resistance is permanent and irreversible (13).

Originally all tubercle bacilli isolated from patients were susceptible to streptomycin, but now 2 or 3 per cent of new cases are due to bacilli which are resistant to streptomycin from the outset. Presumably individuals are being infected by patients who have been treated unsuccessfully with this drug.

Streptomycin produces some toxic manifestations, but these are seldom severe enough or troublesome enough to require that treatment be stopped. In doses of 1 gm daily this drug is reasonably safe, but it is necessary to be familiar with its toxicity. The principal toxic reactions are the following.

1. Damage to the eighth cranial nerve.
2. Renal reactions.
3. Hypersensitivity.
4. Local irritative phenomena.
5. Miscellaneous reactions.

The most common type of toxicity due to streptomycin is its adverse effect on the eighth cranial nerve (14). Both the auditory and the vestibular branches of this nerve may be damaged, but damage to vestibular function is more frequent than auditory damage. Acute vestibular damage is accompanied by headache, vertigo, nausea and vomiting; all of these symptoms are minimal when the patient is at rest, but they are aggravated when he changes position and especially when he attempts coordinated movements. Chronic vestibular damage is not accompanied by headache, nausea or vomiting. In the chronic phase there is vertigo, horizontal nystagmus, ataxia, staggering and even occasional falling. The Romberg test is positive, but the direction is not consistent. There is delay in focusing the eyes; a patient who turns quickly may not be able to focus on objects in his new range of vision for several seconds.

Loss of vestibular function can be demonstrated in the laboratory by the Kobrak caloric test, in which the labyrinth is stimulated by ice water; if there is delay in the onset of nystagmus or reduction in the duration of nystagmus, this is evidence of damaged vestibular function. Damage to the vestibular function is permanent, but the symptoms gradually diminish as the patient compensates for this loss by greater reliance on vision and on deep proprioceptive sensation. In the dark, however, deprived of the help of his vision, the patient with impaired vestibular function continues to experience dizziness, ataxia and some delay in focusing. Usually this does not result in serious disability, but when it is severe, it may interfere with many normal activities.

On doses of 1 gm daily, about 30 per cent of patients become aware of vertigo, and on doses of 1 gm twice a week this is reduced to less than 10 per cent. The incidence of damaged vestibular function as determined by the caloric test is much higher, however. Doses larger than 1 gm daily produce subjective vertigo in almost all patients after a few weeks, and for this reason these large doses are seldom used. The duration of time until vertigo develops varies from case to case, but it usually appears within the first two months of treatment if it appears at all. The mechanism by which damage to vestibular function occurs is not well understood; it may be due to injury to the labyrinth, the vestibular branch of the eighth cranial nerve, or even the vestibular nuclei.

Less common than vestibular damage is damage to the auditory apparatus. The first symptom is tinnitus, which may appear within a week. Tinnitus is a low-pitched, persistant, roaring sound which tends to increase and to lead to deafness if the drug is continued; if the drug is discontinued, tinnitus gradually diminishes over a period of a week or two. Early hearing loss can be recognized only by audiometric examination, since early loss of hearing is usually present in ranges above conversational tones. Hearing loss detectable by audiometry occurs in about 10 per cent of patients who receive streptomycin for long periods of time, but seldom is this loss severe enough to impair hearing in the conversational ranges.

Damage to the auditory function is less important than vestibular damage, since it is less common, and since it usually gives warning by tinnitus when it is impending. However, when it is severe, hearing loss is a great disability. Children and young adults are less likely to suffer hearing loss than older people, and the fetus is even more resistant to this form of streptomycin toxicity, but streptomycin does pass the placental barrier and enter the fetal circulation, and cases are reported of infants who were born with congenital deafness after their mothers had received streptomycin during pregnancy (15). Streptomycin is therefore not the drug of choice in treating tuberculosis in pregnant women.

In an effort to modify streptomycin so as to avoid much of its neurotoxicity, a derivative, dihydrostreptomycin, was prepared. This drug is available as the sulfate. It is more stable than streptomycin, itself, and is very similar to its parent drug in effectiveness against tubercle bacilli. It is absorbed, distributed throughout the body, and excreted in the same way as streptomycin, itself. Dihydrostreptomycin has the advantage that it is far less toxic for the vestibular apparatus; loss of vestibular function occurs later and is less severe with dihydrostreptomycin than with streptomycin. For a time, therefore, dihydrostreptomycin enjoyed great favor. It has been found, however, that this form of the drug has a potentiality for causing serious and progressive deafness. Severe impairment of hearing may result from the use of as little as 5 gm of dihydrostreptomycin. This impairment may be delayed for several weeks or several months, may progress to total deafness and is usually permanent. This ototoxicity is not common but it is severe, unpredictable, and has no warning signs or symptons. Consequently dihydrostreptomycin is now rarely used in the treatment of tuberculosis. A combination of streptomycin and dihydrostreptomycin containing 0.5 gm of each drug has been prepared in the hope that it would be as effective as either drug alone, and that the toxicity would be reduced, but it has been only partially successful. The combination is, in fact, fully effective, its toxicity for the vestibular apparatus is less than that of streptomycin, and its toxicity for the auditory apparatus is less than that of dihydrostreptomycin. Since very small doses of dihydrostreptomycin, as low as a total of 5 gm, have been known to cause progressive and eventually total hearing loss, the bugaboo of total deafness has not been eliminated by the use of this or similar combinations (16). Dihydrostreptomycin, either alone or in combination, is no longer used much in the treatment of tuberculosis.

Renal reactions due to streptomycin are common but seldom serious. Streptomycin may produce tubular irritation, with casts and occasionally albuminuria. Significant impairment of renal function is rare, and when it does occur it almost always clears up promptly when the drug is stopped. Renal damage from streptomycin is thus seen to be rare and usually transient. Preexisting renal disease, however, is a cause for concern in a patient who is receiving streptomycin. Streptomycin is excreted by the kidneys; and if kidney function has been damaged, this excretion may be diminished, and the concentration of the drug in the blood and tissues may rise to toxic levels even though only standard doses have been administered. Tuberculosis of the kidneys is seldom a diffuse disease, so that it seldom damages renal function. Streptomycin is an excellent drug for the treatment of renal tuberculosis, and its use is not attended by any unusual risks.

Hypersensitivity to streptomycin takes many forms, among them eosinophilia, skin rashes, drug fever and joint pain. Hypersensitivity occurs most commonly when large doses are used. Eosinophilia is fairly common, and is not in itself important, but it should alert the physician to watch for other allergic reactions. Skin rashes are of many varieties. The commonest skin reaction is an itchy maculopapular rash which involves most of the body, and may proceed to superficial scaling. Less commonly, there may be urticarial wheals, morbilliform eruptions and even hemorrhagic rashes. Rarely, exfoliative dermatitis occurs, sometimes early in the course of treatment. This explosive antigen-antibody reaction requires immediate cessation of streptomycin treatment, and even then exfoliation may continue for months. Other skin reactions, however, do not necessarily require that the drug be stopped. Antihistaminic drugs help to control the pruritus, and usually the rash subsides even though streptomycin is continued. However, progression of the skin rash or the development of constitutional symptoms require discontinuation of streptomycin treatment. Drug fever is uncommon, and may take two forms, a high sustained fever (102° F to 104° F) or a widely swinging temperature (97° F to 105° F daily). Joint pain is likewise uncommon, and when it occurs it involves usually the small joints of the hands or feet, though any joint may be involved.

When evidence of sensitization exists, it is usually safe to continue streptomycin, except in the case of exfoliative dermatitis. If the drug is stopped because of progression of evidence of hypersensitivity or severity of constitutional reactions, the patient can usually be desensitized by the use of small and gradually ascending doses of streptomycin, so that full doses can be resumed in about a month (17). A suggested desensitization schedule is as follows.

STREPTOMYCIN DESENSITIZATION

Day	Dosage	Day	Dosage	Day	Dosage
1	10 μg	11	1 mg	21	40 mg
2	20 μg	12	1.5 mg	22	60 mg
3	40 μg	13	2 mg	23	100 mg
4	75 μg	14	2.5 mg	24	150 mg
5	100 μg	15	4 mg	25	200 mg
6	200 μg	16	6 mg	26	250 mg
7	300 μg	17	8 mg	27	350 mg
8	450 μg	18	12 mg	28	500 mg
9	600 μg	19	16 mg	29	750 mg
10	750 μg	20	25 mg	30	1000 mg

If hypersensitivity is not severe, desensitization can be accomplished more rapidly. Though continuing streptomycin in the presence of sensitization offers no immediate risk, there is a delayed risk of later development of generalized vascular disease. In these circumstances, the physician must decide whether the advantage of using streptomycin outweighs the possible disadvantages, and may wish to substitute another drug and discontinue streptomycin. However, if no other effective drug is available (because of toxicity, intolerance or bacillary resistance), the risk of delayed vascular damage may be acceptable since it is actually not very great. This decision calls for good clinical judgment.

Hypersensitivity to streptomycin develops not only among patients who receive the drug, but among personnel who prepare and administer it. It is not uncommon in nurses who prepare solutions and administer them to patients. Skin rashes develop, particularly on the hands, and there may be urticaria, asthma, vertigo and eosinophilia. This type of hypersensitivity usually cannot be relieved by desensitization, and the susceptible individual must have no further contact with streptomycin.

There are no cross-immune reactions between streptomycin and dihydrostreptomycin. When there are severe allergic reactions to streptomycin, dihydrostreptomycin may be substituted without fear of similar reactions.

When injected intramuscularly, streptomycin is a moderately irritating drug and dihydrostreptomycin is even more irritating. They produce pain at the site of injection, and sometimes they also produce swelling and induration. These local reactions are usually mild and brief in duration. They are not followed by systemic reactions and they require no treatment. When injected subcutaneously, streptomycin causes a great deal of local pain and irritation. Since subcutaneous injection offers no advantages, this route of administration is rarely used. However, in very thin patients the drug is sometimes deposited subcutaneously by inadvertence, and then the patient suffers considerable discomfort. Intrathecal injection is followed by severe and sometimes serious reactions—headache, nausea, vomiting, local pain, pleocytosis and sometimes root pain and symptoms of irritation of the brain stem (fever, delirium, dyspnoea, bradycardia). Dilute solutions of streptomycin may be injected into the pleural and pericardial cavities and into joint spaces, where they cause only moderate irritation.

There are a few other toxic manifestations which sometimes appear when streptomycin is used. Paresthesias and anesthesias of the lips are fairly common, and so is tingling of the fingertips. There is no pain, and usually the symptoms disappear in a few weeks even if the drug is continued. Streptomycin rarely affects the bone marrow, though leukopenia is occasionally seen. Streptomycin does not damage the liver.

SUMMARY

Streptomycin is an effective antituberculosis drug, considerably less active than isoniazid but nevertheless one of our best drugs. It is given intramuscularly, in doses of 1 gm daily or 1 gm twice weekly, with an effective companion drug. Primary resistance exists in 2 or 3 per cent of cases. Resistance develops in three or four months when streptomycin is used alone, and this brings to an end the usefulness of the drug in that particular case. When used with a companion drug, however, the development of resistance may be delayed for a year or more, providing the opportunity for the disease to become inactive. Streptomycin has a number of toxic manifestations, the most common of which is damage to the eighth cranial nerve. When streptomycin is used, therefore, the patient should be carefully observed and tested for evidence of vestibular or auditory damage, which may require discontinuation of the drug. Other toxic reactions —renal reactions, hypersensitivity, and irritation at the site of injection—seldom require that the drug be stopped. Streptomycin is a valuable antituberculosis drug.

PARA-AMINOSALICYLIC ACID

In 1940, Bernheim noted that benzoic and salicylic acids increase the oxygen consumption of tubercle bacilli. Lehmann explored the effects of a large number of derivatives of benzoic acid, and found that para-aminosalicylic acid (PAS) not only stimulated the oxygen consumption of tubercle bacilli, but that this increased demand for oxygen inhibited both the growth and the multiplication of virulent tubercle bacilli (18). Further studies showed that the administration of PAS by mouth stopped the progression of tuberculosis in guinea-pigs and caused improvement in human tuberculosis (19). The mechanism of this action is uncertain, since there are strains of tubercle bacilli in which PAS does not cause any change in oxidative metabolism, and yet in these strains too, PAS inhibits growth and multiplication.

PAS is a white crystalline powder which is slightly soluble in water but is soluble in alcohol. Aqueous solutions are unstable, darkening and developing an irritating compound (meta-aminophenol) on standing; the same thing is true of the crystalline acid when exposed to moisture, heat or light. It is clear that the acid PAS, though an effective form of the drug, is too unstable to be widely used. Usually one of the salts is used instead. The sodium salt is most generally used, though calcium and potassium salts are also available. The salts are white or cream-colored crystals which are freely soluble in water. PAS is available in many dosage forms.

PAS is rapidly absorbed from the gastrointestinal tract. Following a single dose of 4 gm, the drug reaches a peak concentration of 3 to 12 mg per 100 ml in the blood in one to two hours, and then it disappears rapidly. After it reaches the blood stream, the drug is quickly distributed throughout the total body water, reaching all organs and tissues but penetrating with difficulty into the cerebrospinal fluid. It diffuses readily into caseous masses (20). However, it does not persist long in either normal or tuberculous tissues, but disappears rapidly when the drug is stopped. Within seven hours, 85 per cent of the ingested drug has been excreted by the kidneys, and of this amount more than half appears in the acetylated form (21). Small amounts are excreted in the milk and bile. Sodium PAS and the other salts of PAS are absorbed from the gastrointestinal tract even more rapidly than acid PAS, and reach a peak in the blood more quickly. Thereafter their distribution in the tissues, acetylation, and excretion by the kidneys is identical with that of acid PAS.

The effect of PAS on tubercle bacilli is bacteriostatic. The recommended dose is 12 gm daily, given by mouth in the form of 4 gm three times daily. Because of its irritating effect on the gastric mucosa, it should not be taken fasting, but is best given with meals or immediately after meals. Used as an independent drug in these doses, PAS somewhat retards the progress of human pulmonary tuberculosis and even results in some temporary improvement, but it is of far lower potency than streptomycin or isoniazid. The great value of PAS, however, lies not in its limited usefulness as an independent drug but rather in its use as a companion drug to streptomycin or isoniazid. In culture media, the use of PAS with streptomycin or isoniazid greatly delays the development of resistance to the latter drugs. In experimental animals, these two-drug combinations are far more effective than any single drug. In human tuberculosis, too, the effects of PAS and streptomycin or PAS and isoniazid are synergistic, so that combined therapy is more effective than single-drug therapy. More important, when PAS is used with streptomycin or isoniazid in the treatment of tuberculosis, the development of strains of tubercle bacilli resistant to the major drugs is greatly delayed. This prolongs the duration of effective treatment from a few months to a year or more, and brings about sputum conversion and cavity closure in a high percentage of cases. It is this action of PAS in markedly delaying the development of strains of tubercle bacilli resistant to streptomycin and isoniazid which is its great contribution to the chemotherapy of tuberculosis.

The chief toxic manifestations of PAS are related to the gastro-intestinal tract. A large percentage of patients who take PAS, per-haps a majority, experience some gastrointestinal discomfort, in the form of anorexia, abdominal distention, nausea, vomiting and diar-rhoea. In most cases this is not severe enough to require that the drug be stopped, but in perhaps 10 per cent of patients the symptoms become intolerable and the drug cannot be continued. The very multiplicity of dosage forms—acid PAS, the sodium salt, the calcium salt, the potassium salt, the buffered mixture of acid and sodium PAS (Neopasalate®), the capsules, the enteric-coated granules, the resin-coated granules, the tablets, the enteric-coated tablets, the powders and the solutions—is proof of the fact that many patients have difficulty in taking this drug. The symptoms clear up rapidly when the drug is omitted for a day or two, and often PAS can then be resumed with a lesser degree of intolerance. Sometimes a patient can-not tolerate one dosage form of PAS, but can take another form with a minimum of discomfort. Thus, many who experience great distress on taking the sodium salt of PAS can take the potassium salt or Neopasalate without much difficulty. As has been said before, the irritation of the gastric mucosa can be minimized by ingesting the drug when there is food in the stomach, either during the course of meals or after meals. The taking of milk or antacids just before PAS may be helpful if the drug is to be administered between meals or at bedtime.

Significant allergic reactions occur in about 2.5 per cent of cases receiving PAS (22). Mild forms may begin insidiously with pruritus, a skin rash, a low-grade fever, malaise and eosinophilia. If the drug is not stopped at once, these symptoms may evolve rapidly, so that the patient has high fever, lymphadenopathy, an exfoliative dermatitis, granulocytopenia, encephalopathy and hepatitis with jaundice. Rare-ly, death occurs, usually from fulminating necrosis of the liver (23).

Even mild hypersensitivity reactions demand immediate discontinuation of PAS. A rise in temperature in a patient who was previously afebrile, especially between the second and seventh weeks of treatment, should make one suspicious of hypersensitivity. When combined treatment is being given and hypersensitivity to PAS develops, this is often followed by the development of cross-hypersensitivity to the companion drug as well. If it is important that the patient should receive PAS, desensitization can usually be carried out. Berte *et al* (24), have recommended the following schedule.

ORAL PAS DESENSITIZATION SCHEDULE

(Days 1-12: A 0.1 per cent Solution of Sodium PAS Used)

Days	Amount Given in CC	Dose of PAS in Mg	No. of Doses Daily
1	0.12	0.12	1
2	0.25	0.25	1
3	0.50	0.50	1
4	1	1	1
5	1	1	3
6	2	2	3
7	4	4	3
8	8	8	3
9	15	15	3
10	30	30	3
11	60	60	3
12	100	100	3

(Days 13-24: A 1.0 per cent Solution of Sodium PAS Used)

Days	Amount Given in CC	Dose of PAS in Mg	No. of Doses Daily
13	5	50	3
14	8	80	3
15	10	100	3
16	20	200	3
17	20	200	3
18	40	400	3
19	40	400	3
20	60	600	3
21	60	600	3
22	100	1000	3
23	100	1000	3
24	100	1000	3

(Days 25-34: Weighed Sodium PAS Powder Used)

Days	Dose of PAS in Gm	No. of Doses Daily
25	1	3
26	1	3
27	1	3
28	2	3
29	2	3
30	2	3
31	3	3
32	3	3
33	3	3
34	4	3

However, there is some risk of a repetition of the reaction or of the later development of generalized vascular disease. If a satisfactory secondary drug is available, it is usually safest to discontinue PAS and substitute another drug.

An alternate method of coping with hypersensitivity to PAS, if it is important to continue the drug, is to administer the adrenocorticosteroid hormones along with it. Using this technique, one administers 30 to 60 mg of prednisone or its equivalent the first day and then reduces the dose gradually to 20 mg daily; this dose is continued for about four weeks and is then tapered off and discontinued. While the steroid is being given, rapid desensitization to PAS can be carried out safely, going from 0.5 gm three times daily to four gm three times daily in about a week.

An uncommon reaction to PAS is the development of goiter (25), which is caused by the blocking of iodine accumulation in the thyroid by the drug. This does not require discontinuation of treatment. The thyroid returns to normal when PAS is stopped.

Patients who are on low sodium diets should obviously not receive any form of PAS which contains sodium, such as sodium PAS or Neopasalate, since these contain large amounts of sodium. These patients should receive their PAS in some other form, such as the calcium or potassium salts or Neopasalate-K.

Primary resistance to PAS is rare (26), and is in all cases probably due to infection by patients who had been treated unsuccessfully with PAS. When treated with PAS alone, patients rarely convert their sputum, and the tubercle bacilli eventually become resistant, but at a slower rate than occurs with streptomycin or isoniazid. This development of resistance to PAS when the drug is used alone is now only of historical interest, since this drug is never used alone. When used as a companion to another drug, resistance to both PAS and the other drug is greatly delayed (27), and usually the sputum becomes negative before resistant strains develop. Tubercle bacilli resistant to PAS in the test tube are also resistant in the animal body and in human patients.

Summary

Para-aminosalicylic acid (PAS), in doses of 4 gm three times daily by mouth, is a tuberculostatic drug of rather feeble potency. It

has one great value. When it is given as a companion drug to streptomycin or isoniazid, it delays for a long time the development of resistance to those drugs, thereby greatly increasing the duration of
their effectiveness as antituberculosis drugs. This permits drug treatment to be definitive treatment, capable of rendering the sputum negative and of allowing cavities to close and heal without resectional
surgery. When surgery is necessary, combined therapy permits it tc
be done with a minimum of tuberculous complications. PAS tends
to irritate the gastorintestinal tract, producing anorexia, nausea, vomiting and diarrhoea. However, in only about 10 per cent of patients
are these symptoms severe enough to require abandonment of treatment. Severe allergic reactions occur in about 2.5 per cent of patients,
and these require that the drug be stopped immediately.

Though of only slight tuberculostatic power when used alone, PAS
is considered a first-line drug because of its great value as a companion drug to streptomycin and isoniazid. When used with these
drugs it greatly increases their effectiveness and prolongs their usefulness.

REFERENCES

1. SELIKOFF, I. J., AND ROBITZEK, E. K.: Tuberculosis chemotherapy
   with hydrazine derivatives of isonicotinic acid. *Dis. Chest, 21*:385,
   1952.

2. ELMENDORF, D. G., CAWTHON, W. U., MUSCHENHEIM, C., AND
   McDERMOTT, W.: Absorption, distribution, excretion, and short-
   term toxicity of isonicotinic acid hydrazide in man. *Amer. Rev.
   Tuberc., 65*:429, 1952.

3. MANTHEI, R. W., ROTH, L. J., BARCLAY, W. R., AND EBERT, R. H.:
   The distribution of C^{14}-labelled isoniazid in tissues and body
   fluids of tuberculous patients and guinea pigs. *Trans. twelfth
   conference chemotherapy tuberculosis,* p. 245, 1953.

4. BROMBERG, Y. M., SALZBERGER, M., AND BRUDERMAN, I.: Placental
   transmission of isonicotinic acid hydrazide. *Gynaecologia, 140*:3,
   1955.

5. POPE, H.: The neutralization of isoniazid activity in M. tuberculosis
   by certain metabolites. *Amer. Rev. Tuberc., 73*:735, 1956.

6. BIEHL, J. P., AND NIMITZ, H. J.: Studies on the use of a high dosage
   of isoniazid. *Amer. Rev. Tuberc., 70*:430, 1954.

7. Biehl, J. P., and Vilter, R. W.: Effects of isoniazid on pyridoxine metabolism. *JAMA, 156*:1549, 1954.

8. Hobby, G. L.: Primary drug resistance in tuberculosis. *Amer. Rev. Resp. Dis., 87*:29, 1963.

9. Schatz, A., Bugie, E., and Waksman, S. A.: Streptomycin substance exhibiting antibiotic activity against gram-positive and gram-negative bacteria. *Proc. Soc. Exp. Biol. Med., 55*:66, 1944.

10. Rake, G., and Donovick, R., Absorption distribution, and excretion of streptomycin. In *Streptomycin*, edited by Waksman, S. A., Baltimore, Williams and Wilkins, 1949.

11. Smith, K. M.: Miliary and meningeal tuberculosis. *Minutes of the eighth streptomycin conference*, p. 165, 1949.

12. Smith, K. M.: "Assorted" tuberculosis, summary discussion. *Minutes of the eighth streptomycin conference*, p. 170, 1949.

13. Yegian, D., and Vanderlinde, R. J.: The resistance of tubercle bacilli to chemotherapeutic agents. *Amer. Rev. Tuberc., 61*:483, 1950.

14. Cooper, D. A.: Toxicity of streptomycin. *Trans. tenth conference chemotherapy tuberculosis*, p. 217, 1951.

15. Robinson, G. C., and Cambon, K. G.: Hearing loss in infants of tuberculous mothers treated with streptomycin during pregnancy. *New Eng. J. Med., 271*:949, 1964.

16. Glorig, A.: The effect of dihydrostreptomycin hydrochloride and sulfate on the auditory mechanism. *Ann. Otol., 60*:327, 1951.

17. Cohen, A. C., and Glinsky, G. C.: Hypersensitivity to streptomycin. *J. Allerg., 22*:63, 1951.

18. Lehmann, I.: Para-aminosalicylic acid in treatment of tuberculosis. *Lancet, 1*:15, 1946.

19. The therapeutic trials committee of the Swedish National Association against tuberculosis, para-aminosalicylic acid treatment in pulmonary tuberculosis. *Amer. Rev. Tuberc., 61*:597, 1950.

20. Heller, A., Ebert, R. H., Koch-Weser, D., and Roth, L. J.: Studies with C[14]-labelled para-aminosalicylic acid and isoniazid. *Amer. Rev. Tuberc., 75*:71, 1957.

21. Way, E. L., Smith, P. K., Howie, D. L., Weiss, R., and Swanson, R.: The absorption, distribution, excretion and fate of para-aminosalicylic acid. *J. Pharmacol. Exp. Ther., 93*:368, 1948.

22. Alt, W. J., and Spengler, J. R.: Severe systemic reactions to para-aminosalicylic acid. *Ann. Intern. Med., 45*:541, 1956.

23. Hansen, J. E., and Cleve, E. A.: Fatal hypersensitivity to PAS and streptomycin. *Dis. Chest., 28*:577, 1955.

24. BERTE, S. J., DI MASE, J. D., AND CHRISTIANSON, C. S.: Isoniazid, para-aminosalicyclic acid, and streptomycin intolerance in 1744 patients, Personal communication.

25. BRINKMAN, G. L., AND COATES, E. O.: The goitrogenic effect of para-aminosalicylic acid during the therapy of pulmonary tuberculosis. *Amer. Rev. Tuberc., 69*:458, 1954.

26. DYE, W. E.: Para-aminosalicylic acid resistant M. tuberculosis. U. S. Armed Forces Med. Jour., *1*:1137, 1950.

27. GRAESSLE, O. E., AND PIETROWSKI, J. J.: The *in vitro* effect of p-aminosalicylic acid in preventing acquired resistance to streptomycin by M. tuberculosis. *J. Bact., 57*:459, 1949.

Chapter V

THE SECONDARY DRUGS

ETHIONAMIDE

Ethionamide is a drug with a chemical structure closely related to that of isoniazid. It is 2-ethyl-thioisonicotinamide, like isoniazid, a derivative of isonicotinic acid. It was developed in the course of a search for an antituberculosis drug effective against bacilli which were resistant to isoniazid, streptomycin and PAS. In this search, a series of isonicotinic acid derivatives was examined, and in 1956, ethionamide was found to meet the requirements (1). It is a yellow, crystalline compound, almost insoluble in water and ether but freely soluble in ethyl alcohol. After being taken by mouth, it is absorbed slowly from the gut, and suppositories yield an even slower absorption rate. Once absorbed, it is rapidly and widely distributed throughout the body, the concentration in serum and organs being approximately identical (2). Following oral administration, the maximum blood level is reached in about three hours (3). Both in normal individuals and in patients with meningitis, ethionamide reaches a peak concentration in the cerebrospinal fluid about three hours after ingestion (4). The drug is eliminated from the body more rapidly than isoniazid. It is excreted by the kidneys (5). In one of the metabolic pathways of ethionamide, the drug is methylated and then oxidized to N'-methyl-pyridone, in which form it is excreted in the urine (6).

Since ethionamide is adequately absorbed from the gut, the oral route is the one which is almost always used, though the drug can also be administered in the form of suppositories. The optimum dose is the highest tolerated dose, and in most people this is 0.5 gm twice daily.

Though less effective than isoniazid, ethionamide is a useful antituberculosis drug. It is fully active against tubercle bacilli which are

resistant to isoniazid, streptomycin (7), PAS, viomycin and cycloserine, and has proven effective in infections due to unclassified mycobacteria. In human tuberculosis, the optimum dose is 0.5 gm twice
daily, given by mouth. If this dose cannot be tolerated, lesser doses,
0.25 gm twice or three times daily, are often adequate. Because of
possible gastrointestinal intolerance, it is best to start with the dose
of 0.25 gm twice daily, and increase this by 0.25 gm daily each week
for two weeks, unless prevented by gastric symptoms, so that the full
dose of 0.5 gm twice weekly is reached over a period of two weeks.
On this dosage the clinical response in previously untreated cases is
good (8), but not as good as we have come to expect from isoniazid.
Fever subsides, sputum volume diminishes, the sputum becomes negative, and there is clearing by x-ray and sometimes cavity closure,
but the improvement is slower and less complete than when isoniazid
is used. There seems, therefore, to be no advantage to using this
drug instead of isoniazid in previously untreated cases.

Ethionamide has its greatest field of usefulness in chronic pulmonary
tuberculosis due to tubercle bacilli resistant to streptomycin and
isoniazid. Used with a second drug to which the bacilli are susceptible, significant clinical and radiological improvement occurs in a
majority of cases, the sputum becomes negative in a good number
(9), and, in a smaller number, resectional surgery becomes possible.
In this very difficult group of patients, who have failed to recover on
treatment with the first-line drugs, this degree of improvement is a
worthwhile accomplishment.

The toxicity of ethionamide is considerable, and requires discontinuation of treatment in about 30 per cent of cases. Most common
are gastrointestinal complaints, which occur to some extent in the
great majority of cases (8). Most patients experience nausea, anorexia and weight loss, and many have a metallic taste in the mouth,
salivation, gastric pain and burning, vomiting and diarrhoea (10).
Usually these symptoms are not severe enough to require cessation of
treatment, and they usually diminish after a few weeks but do not
entirely disappear. Some patients complain of peripheral neuropathy
(10) (11), which may be severe and prolonged. Generally, however, the nerve pain disappears when administration of the drug is
stopped. Since the neuropathy is often associated with gastrointestinal

complaints, it may be pellagrous in nature, and should be treated not only with pyridoxine but with other elements of the vitamin B complex. Gynecomastia, photodermatitis, and mental confusion are less common toxic manifestations (10). Though not common, liver damage is the most serious form of toxicity to ethionamide (8) (10) (12) (13). About 10 per cent of patients who receive ethionamide develop evidence of abnormal liver function, and 1 per cent or more develop frank jaundice. All in all, while the toxic manifestations of ethionamide are seldom serious, in about 30 per cent of cases they are unpleasant enough and persistent enough to require discontinuation of the drug.

Ethionamide is usually fully effective against tubercle bacilli which are resistant to isoniazid, streptomycin and other drugs. Only the thiosemicarbazones exhibit cross-resistance with ethionamide. However, primary resistance to ethionamide does occur, sometimes to a slight degree and sometimes to a degree so great that clinical benefit is unlikely to result from its use. When the tubercle bacilli are initially susceptible, resistance develops quickly when the drug is given alone, but it develops slowly if an effective companion drug is used.

Summary

Ethionamide is a useful antituberculosis drug, being not quite as effective as streptomycin. Its optimum dosage is 0.5 gm twice daily, though smaller doses (0.25 gm twice daily) are also effective. In full doses the majority of patients experience gastrointestinal intolerance, and there are other toxic manifestations, the most serious of which is hepatitis. Because of its toxicity, ethionamide is not suitable for the initial therapy of tuberculosis. Since it is usually fully effective against tubercle bacilli which are resistant to isoniazid and streptomycin, its greatest usefulness is in the treatment of tuberculosis due to bacilli resistant to these drugs.

PYRAZINAMIDE

Pyrazinamide (pyrazinoic acid amide) is chemically related to the thiosemicarbazones. It is a white crystalline powder, stable indefinitely

at room temperature, and soluble in water. It is readily absorbed
following oral administration, reaches effective levels in the blood and
tissues, and is excreted by the kidneys. Pyrazinamide is an antibacterial agent useful in the treatment of tuberculosis. It is an effective
secondary drug. It is given by mouth, and the adult dose is 0.5 gm
to 1 gm three times daily. When given with isoniazid, its antituberculosis activity is very great; in mice this combination appears to eradi-
cate tuberculosis entirely from the animal tissues (14), and in man
this combination is therapeutically equal or superior to isoniazid and
PAS (15). The optimum dose is 50 mg per kg.

Pyrazinamide produces toxic manifestations of several varieties. The
most common and the most important is toxic hepatitis (16). This
occurs in about 15 per cent of patients who receive this drug. It may
occur at any time during the course of treatment—as early as the
seventeenth day, and as late as the eighth month—and does not
appear to be related to dose, occurring about as often at doses of
0.5 gm three times daily as at doses of 1 gm three times daily. The
earliest evidence of liver damage is usually elevation of the enzyme
serum glutamic oxalacetic transaminase, while an increase of the
bromsulfalein retention is more significant evidence of liver toxicity.
The incidence of jaundice is about 3 or 4 per cent, and some deaths
have occurred (17). Liver toxicity is more common in older than
in younger patients, but it is not limited to patients with previously
damaged livers. If pyrazinamide is stopped at the first evidence of
liver damage, there is no progression of this damage, and the liver
function gradually returns to normal. Liver biopsy shows that the
structural damage to the liver takes the form of widely distributed
areas of focal necrosis. In fulminating cases, the time between onset
of symptoms and death may be only a few days, and the entire archi-
tecture of the liver may be destroyed. Because of the occasional
severe damage to the liver, pyrazinamide is too dangerous to be used
in the original treatment of patients with tuberculosis, even under
close observation in a hospital. When it is used in patients who have
failed to recover on treatment with the primary drugs, the patient
should be closely observed for evidence of hepatitis—jaundice, liver
enlargement, liver tenderness—and should have frequent determina-
tions of the bromsulfalein retention and the serum glutamic oxalacetic
transaminase.

The other toxic manifestations of pyrazinamide are not serious. Pyrazinamide increases reabsorption of urates in the renal tubules, causing the serum uric acid to rise; levels of 9 mg per 100 ml are common, and levels as high as 15 mg per 100 ml are not unusual. Probenecid sometimes reduces the hyperuricemic effect of pyrazinamide, but this is not dependable. Following prolonged use of pyrazinamide, clinical gouty arthritis develops in a small number of patients, about five per thousand. This can be treated satisfactorily with colchicine, and does not require that the drug be stopped (18). Following withdrawal of the drug the uric acid levels in most cases return to their previous range within forty-eight hours. Other side effects which sometimes occur are arthralgia, anorexia and malaise; these are mild, and do not interfere with the treatment.

When pyrazinamide is used alone, there is initial improvement followed by deterioration which begins in from one to three months. The laboratory determination of resistance to pyrazinamide is unreliable, but the early deterioration is believed to be due to the development of resistant organisms. When used with isoniazid or another companion drug, the development of resistance to both pyrazinamide and the companion drug is delayed, so that there is a longer period of clinical usefulness.

Summary

Pyrazinamide is an effective secondary antituberculosis drug. Used with isoniazid, the combination is extremely effective in mice, and is at least as effective as isoniazid and PAS in human tuberculosis. It is capable of causing severe damage to the liver, and is therefore too dangerous to be used in the original treatment of patients with tuberculosis. However, when treatment with the basic drugs has failed, pyrazinamide may be a very satisfactory drug to employ. When it is used, the patient should be closely observed for evidence of hepatitis.

CYCLOSERINE

Cycloserine is an antibiotic derived from Streptomyces orchidaceus. It is a white crystalline powder, freely soluble in water and hygroscopic; it gradually loses potency when exposed to heat or light. It is rapidly and totally absorbed from the upper gastrointestinal tract, so that the bacterial flora of the lower intestines is not modified (19).

Two hours after the ingestion of 250 mg of the drug, its concentration in the serum often reaches 15 to 30 μg per ml, though there is no consistent relationship between dosage and blood levels. The concentration in lung tissue exceeds that in the blood, and the concentration in the pleural fluid, cerebrospinal fluid, milk and fetal blood are about the same as that found in the patient's blood. Appreciable amounts are also found in all the organs (20), and in the bile and sputum. About 50 per cent of the ingested drug is excreted in the urine in twenty-four hours, and about 65 per cent in seventy-two hours; the remaining 35 per cent is apparently metabolized to unknown substances (21).

In concentrations of 10 μg per ml cycloserine causes partial to complete inhibition of the growth of virulent tubercle bacilli in a liquid medium in the test tube (22). Clinically, this concentration can be attained readily, usually by using a dosage of 250 mg twice daily or oftener. The drug is fully effective against strains of tubercle bacilli which are resistant to streptomycin and and isoniazid (23). As a dependable tuberculostatic drug, cycloserine is less active than isoniazid or streptomycin, but it is effective enough to make it a useful drug. There is no evidence of antagonism to other antituberculosis drugs, so it may be used in any combination. Given as the sole drug, there is usually temporary clinical improvement, and the progression of tuberculosis stops; however, the improvement is transient, since resistance develops rapidly. Used with a companion drug to which the bacilli are susceptible, cycloserine usually remains effective for a good many months, and a good result is often obtained. Since most of the toxicity of cycloserine is neurologic or psychiatric, and since it has been shown that on doses greater than 0.8 gm per day there is a great increase in the urinary excretion of pyridoxine, it has been recommended that pyridoxine in doses up to 300 mg daily be administered when cycloserine is used. This not only reduces its toxicity, but as a result it permits larger and more effective doses to be given.

Cycloserine is definitely not a first-line drug. Its toxicity and its limited effectiveness in low doses make its use unwise in original-treatment cases. However, used with another drug to which the tubercle bacilli are susceptible, and used in full doses, it is very helpful in the treatment of patients who have failed to recover on the basic drugs and whose bacilli have become resistant to them (24). In this group of patients, doses of 500 mg to 2000 mg daily are needed. It is desirable to attain serum concentrations of 25 μg per ml or higher. A satisfactory regimen is to start with 250 mg every twelve hours, and to add 250 mg daily every ten days until the patient is receiving 2 gm daily in about two months. In this hard-core group of patients it is not common to see much improvement by x-ray, though progression of disease stops and there may be some resolution of exudative lesions. There is good clinical improvement, though, and reduction of the sputum volume. Above all, there is frequently conversion of the sputum, and sometimes, even in these old chronic cases, the disease is stabilized and resection of troublesome residual cavitary disease becomes possible (25). In large doses, the combination of cycloserine and a companion drug is sometimes impressively effective; large cavities which have been producing positive sputum for several years often cease to produce positive sputum, and sometimes when these cavities are resected they prove to have undergone open healing.

Toxicity limits the use of cycloserine. The toxic manifestations are principally neurologic or psychiatric. These neuropsychiatric disturbances cannot be predicted. They are not related to age, sex or duration of tuberculosis. It is impossible to establish any valid correlation between the clinical toxic manifestations and disturbances of the electroencephalograms (26). It is probably wise not to give the drug to patients who have a history of epilepsy or psychosis. Neurological effects include muscular weakness, tremors, increased reflexes, ankle clonus, ataxia, slurred speech, blurred vision and convulsions. The psychic effects include nervousness, insomnia, restlessness, somnolence, increased libido, anxiety, inability to concentrate, loss of judgment, a tendency to impulsive behavior, lapses of memory, confusion, delusions and hallucinations. Some patients become suspicious and some become frankly paranoid. Suicidal ideas have been expressed, and a few patients have actually committed suicide. The use of pyridoxine, anti-convulsants, and tranquillizers greatly reduces the frequency and severity of the neurological complications, but the psychiatric toxicity is much more difficult to cope with. If significant psychic side effects occur, it is best to discontinue cycloserine; once the drug has been stopped the side effects usually disappear promptly. However, some of the paranoid reactions have persisted for a long time.

Primary drug resistance is not infrequent in the case of cycloserine.

Resistance to 10 μg per ml is not at all uncommon, and some strains of tubercle bacilli resistant to as much as 50 μg per ml have been isolated from patients who have never been treated with this antibiotic (27). These resistant strains are fully virulent for experimental animals and men. Organisms resistant to 10 μg per ml do not pose a serious therapeutic problem, since concentrations higher than this can readily be attained in the blood. However, tubercle bacilli resistant to 25 μg per ml or more will not respond to therapy with cycloserine, since in these cases adequate concentrations of the drug in the tissues cannot be attained. If cycloserine is given alone to patients infected with cycloserine-susceptible tubercle bacilli, these bacilli will quickly become resistant. If cycloserine is given with an effective companion drug, resistance to cycloserine develops much more slowly, and it protects its companion drug against the development of resistance too. In the latter respect, though, cycloserine is not as good as PAS in delaying the development of resistance to the second drug.

Summary

Cycloserine is a useful antituberculosis drug, less valuable than streptomycin or isoniazid but distinctly helpful. Its value is limited by its toxicity, which principally affects the neuropsychiatric system. This toxicity is formidable, and its manifestations include convulsions and psychoses. However, the neurological complications can be minimized by the use of tranquillizers, anti-convulsants and pyridoxine, and the psychic complications are usually transient if the drug is stopped as soon as they become manifest. Cycloserine should not be used if the tubercle bacilli are susceptible to isoniazid, streptomycin and PAS. When dealing with disease due to tubercle bacilli resistant to these basic drugs, cycloserine is a useful secondary drug.

ETHAMBUTOL

Ethambutol is still in the investigational stage. It shows great promise, but it is not yet on the market.

Ethambutol is the dextrorotatory form of 2, 2', (ethylene—diimine) -di-1-butanol. The levorotatory form is inactive against mycobacteria and is equally toxic. Ethambutol is a white crystalline powder, soluble in water, and heat-stable. In the test tube it inhibits the growth of tubercle bacilli in concentrations of 1 to 4 μg per ml (28) (29). It is fully effective against bacilli which are resistant to streptomycin, isoniazid, ethionamide and kanamycin, and is also active against many unclassified mycobacteria. When taken by mouth, the drug is rapidly absorbed from the gastrointestinal tract, and is present in maximal concentration in the serum in one to two hours. Serum concentrations are proportional to the dose administered. A dose of 25 mg per kg body weight produces a peak serum level of about 5 μg per ml, while a dose of 50 mg per kg yields a peak serum level of about 10 μg per ml. The serum concentration drops rapidly, so that twenty-four hours after the ingestion of an oral dose the serum level is only about 10 per cent of the peak concentration. The drug is rapidly excreted in the urine. In patients receiving ethambutol daily, more than 50 per cent is excreted unchanged in the urine within twenty-four hours (30), in addition to a further quantity which is excreted in the form of metabolites (31). When doses of 25 mg per kg or 50 mg per kg are employed, there is no accumulation of ethambutol in the body, but when larger doses are used there may be some accumulation.

Ethambutol is an effective drug in both human and animal tuberculosis. In doses of 100 mg per kg, it produces results about as good as those achieved by isoniazid in optimum doses. Because of toxicity this dose level is seldom used. In the usual dosage of 25 mg per kg ethambutol is inferior to isoniazid; it produces good clearing of the pulmonary lesions, but the clearing is neither as prompt nor as complete as that produced by isoniazid in adequate doses. However, though one of the tests of a drug's value is its effectiveness when used alone, antituberculosis drugs are seldom used alone. Used in combination with isoniazid, even small doses of ethambutol increase the therapeutic effectiveness of the regimen and retard the development of bacilli resistant to isoniazid (32). The same thing is true when ethambutol is used in combination with other drugs such as pyrazinamide, cycloserine, streptomycin, PAS, ethionamide or viomycin. Even in the difficult-to-treat patients who have failed to recover on the basic drugs and some of the secondary drugs, combinations using ethambutol almost always produce symptomatic benefit, often result in clearing of the pulmonary lesions, and not infrequently convert the sputum to negative. The drug is readily accepted by patients, having no unpleasant taste and no gastrointestinal side effects (33) (34).

It is clear that its effectiveness could make ethambutol a very helpful antituberculosis drug, but its usefulness is limited by its toxicity. In monkeys, doses of less than 400 mg per kg, and serum levels of less than 20 μg per ml, have failed to produce significant toxicity. Since doses of 25 mg to 100 mg per kg and serum levels of 2 μg per ml have been shown to be effective, there seems to be a wide margin of safety. When doses of 400 mg per kg and higher are given to monkeys, lesions of the central nervous system often develop. These lesions have been found in the optic chiasm and optic tracts, in the midbrain, in the pyramidal tracts, and in the cervical cord. Microscopically there is swelling and dissolution of myelin and degeneration and necrosis of nerve cells accompanied by glial proliferation. The monkeys which receive doses of 800 mg per kg or more for several months regularly develop symptoms of central nervous system dysfunction. These symptoms include ataxia, muscular weakness, loss of grasping reflexes, loss of vision, and labored breathing which is asthmatic in type. Ethambutol causes no toxic reactions in any organs other than the central nervous system in monkeys (32). In dogs, doses of 400 mg per kg, per day, produce changes in the heart muscle, and sometimes death from myocardial failure. Ethambutol sometimes produces optic toxicity in human beings even in doses of 25 mg per kg; up to the present time the damage to vision has always been transient, but it is unpleasant and rather frightening while it lasts, and recovery may be slow. The early symptoms of visual damage are blurring and hazy vision. This is followed by progressive decrease in visual acuity, contraction of the visual fields, central scotomas, and poor color discrimination. Ethambutol causes no damage to kidney function, liver function, or the blood-forming organs, but one asthmatic patient is reported to have died in typical status asthmaticus (33).

Primary resistance to ethambutol has not been reported. When given in combination with other drugs, resistance to ethambutol develops slowly, and the development of resistance to the second drug is greatly delayed. As a result, the benefits of this drug in combined therapy may be expected to be long-lasting.

Summary

Ethambutol is effective in the treatment of tuberculosis even when the bacilli are resistant to streptomycin, isoniazid, ethionamide and kanamycin. In combination with other drugs it can be helpful in the management of disease due to resistant tubercle bacilli. Its central nervous system toxicity, resulting in severe damage to monkeys in large doses, and in visual loss in man in doses as low as 25 mg per kg, limits its usefulness. For the present, its principal use is in the treatment of tuberculosis due to bacilli resistant to the basic drugs. In such cases it may be used in doses of 25 mg per kg for a relatively short time, for example, as coverage for surgery, or it may be used for longer periods in smaller doses. It is being used experimentally as a second drug, with isoniazid or streptomycin, in the treatment of patients who have never received antituberculosis drugs previously. For this purpose the recommended dosage is 25 mg per kg for two months, then 15 mg per kg. In these doses no clinical toxicity has been reported.

More effective than PAS, and better tolerated by patients, it may turn out to be the best adjunct to isoniazid or streptomycin in the primary treatment of tuberculosis, but much more experience is needed as to its toxicity before it is widely used. Whenever ethambutol is used visual field examinations should be performed every two weeks, and treatment should be stopped if there are complaints of visual disturbances or evidence of contraction of the visual fields.

CAPREOMYCIN

Capreomycin is another promising antituberculosis drug which has been available for study for several years, but which is not yet on the market.

Capreomycin is an antibiotic produced by Streptomyces capreolus. It is highly soluble in water, is stable in the middle p^H ranges, has been shown to be a peptide including the amino-acids alanine, serine, betalysine, as well as several others. It has a molecular weight of 740. It is active in the test tube against several species of mycobacteria, including the tubercle bacillus and M.kansasii. It is effective in the treatment of tuberculous infection in mice (35). In man, when capreomycin is injected intramuscularly, it is absorbed rapidly, and then is gradually excreted by the kidneys. Following intramuscular injections, a considerable amount of the drug appears in the blood stream in half an hour and peak blood level is reached in one hour. Good blood levels are maintained for only two or three hours, and then they drop rapidly. In eight hours approximately half of the capreomycin has been excreted in the urine. At the end of twenty-four hours there is usually no detectable capreomycin in the blood, and there is no significant accumulation in the blood when the drug is given in doses of 1 gm daily.

The optimum dose in man is 1 gm daily, given intramuscularly. In human tuberculosis, capreomycin has been used both in patients who have had no previous drug treatment and in those who have had treatment with other drugs but who have failed to improve or have relapsed. Capreomycin has been shown to be a valuable drug, perhaps a little less effective than streptomycin and much less effective than isoniazid but still a worthwhile addition to our armamentarium. At present its greatest field of usefulness is in the treatment of those patients whose tubercle bacilli are resistant to streptomycin, PAS and isoniazid; capreomycin is fully effective against such bacilli (35) (36). There is no incompatibility between this drug and any other antituberculosis drug, so that it can be used in any combination. However, it should not be used with streptomycin, viomycin or kanamycin, even if these drugs have not been rendered useless by the emergence of bacilli resistant to them, because their toxicity is similar to that of capreomycin, and the combined toxicity might be extremely damaging.

The toxicity of capreomycin is not great, and is almost entirely limited to the kidneys and the eighth cranial nerve (36). In the kidneys, capreomycin tends to damage the tubular epithelium. This occurs fairly common in animal experiments, and in many the PSP excretion, which is a test of renal tubular function, is often decreased both at fifteen minutes and at sixty minutes after injection of the dye. In one human case, there was definite tubular damage which somewhat resembled the damage caused by mercury bichloride. There are also reports of elevation of the blood urea nitrogen and nonprotein nitrogen. The sequence of events is that capreomycin may cause significant injury to the renal tubules, and when tubular excretion is interfered with there is likely to be a rise in the blood urea nitrogen and nonprotein nitrogen.

Another consequence of impaired tubular excretion is that serum levels of capreomycin may rise dangerously. Fortunately capreomycin does not often injure the renal tubular epithelium, but since such injury may evolve rapidly and become a serious threat in a short time tests of kidney function must be done at frequent intervals when this drug is being administered. Urinalysis and either the blood urea nitrogen or the nonprotein nitrogen should be done every two weeks, and the PSP excretion test should be done monthly, when capreomycin is being given. If there is any evidence of significant damage of renal function, the drug should be discontinued.

Hearing loss has been reported, but is not common, occurring in about 3 per cent of patients who receive capreomycin in full doses. It appears to be permanent, but is not complete and does not progress after treatment is discontinued. When it is detected the drug should be stopped, because continuation of capreomycin in these circumstances is likely to cause further deterioration of hearing. Capreomycin causes little impairment of vestibular function, though some patients complain of dizziness, and asymptomatic decrease of vestibular function has been reported.

There is a wide variety of other toxic manifestations which are either unimportant or rare. Several animals receiving capreomycin have developed cataracts. Though the mechanism is not understood and no cases are known to have occurred in man, regular examinations of the eye are recommended in patients who are taking capreomycin. There have been a number of minor complaints, such as dizziness, tingling of the fingers or face, skin rashes and vague aches and pains. These are usually inconsequential and transient. Animal reproduction studies are not yet reported, and until these are available, capreomycin should not be given to pregnant women or to any woman of child-bearing age.

Drug fever has occasionally been reported, and is usually a contraindication to further use of the drug. No other allergic manifestations to capreomycin are known, either among patients who have received the drug or among personnel who have handled it (37).

Initial resistance to capreomycin does not exist. Cross resistance with isoniazid, streptomycin, kanamycin or other drugs, does not exist; small doses of capreomycin will inhibit the growth of organisms which are highly resistant to these drugs. Tubercle bacilli do become resistant to capreomycin after prolonged exposure to it, either in the test tube or in animals or man, but resistance is slow in developing. When resistance develops, the drug has lost its effectiveness. With capreomycin, as with streptomycin, resistance in the test tube parallels clinical resistance.

Summary

Capreomycin is a moderately effective drug, less effective than isoniazid but of the same order of value as streptomycin. It is given intramuscularly in doses of 1 gm daily. Its toxicity is not great, and is principally limited to the kidneys and the eighth cranial nerve. Capreomycin is capable of injuring the tubular epithelium of the kidneys, and when this happens the drug should be discontinued. Hearing loss also occurs occasionally, and this too requires that the drug be stopped. Initial resistance does not occur; resistance may develop as a result of treatment, but it develops slowly. Capreomycin is a worthwhile addition to our armamentarium; its greatest value is in the treatment of patients whose disease is due to streptomycin-resistant bacilli.

VIOMYCIN

Viomycin is an antibiotic obtained from the actinomycete Streptomyces puniceus. It is a strongly basic substance which is available as the sulfate, a white or pale yellow crystalline powder freely soluble in water. This powder is stable at room temperature for as long as two years. Aqueous solutions are stable for one week at temperatures of $2°$ to $10°$ C, but are inactivated by heat. Viomycin sulfate is poorly absorbed from the gastrointestinal tract. Following intramuscular injection, the drug is rapidly absorbed, and it soon appears in the serum in concentrations higher than needed to inhibit tubercle bacilli. Small concentrations appear in the cerebrospinal fluid and in the pleural and peritoneal cavities. Viomycin is excreted by the kidneys, 65 to 100 per cent of an injected dose appearing in the urine within twenty-four hours (38).

Viomycin in doses of 2 gm twice weekly is active against tubercle bacilli whether they are susceptible or resistant to streptomycin or isoniazid. Concentrations of 5 μg per ml completely inhibit the growth of tubercle bacilli. Viomycin is very active in retarding the progress of tuberculosis in guinea pigs, 40 mg viomycin having activity equal to 10 mg of streptomycin. It is less effective than isoniazid or streptomycin (39) (40), but is nevertheless a drug of considerable value. Because of its toxicity it should not be used in the treatment of patients whose tubercle bacilli are susceptible to the usual drugs. It should always be used in conjunction with a second effective drug, and the second drug should not be streptomycin because the toxicity of the two drugs is so similar. The combinations, cycloserine and viomycin or pyrazinamide and viomycin are often used successfully.

Toxic manifestations very similar to those of streptomycin are common, occurring in about half of all patients who receive viomycin. Most toxicity is minor and transient, so that treatment does not have to be interrupted or dosage reduced, but in more than 10 per cent of cases the drug cannot be tolerated and the treatment must be stopped. Most patients complain that viomycin causes pain and tenderness at the site of injection, and some develop induration. Care should be taken to see that the injections are always given intramuscularly, since viomycin is quite irritating if it is given subcutaneously by mistake. Impairment of function of the eighth cranial nerve is quite common. Many patients notice vertigo, and caloric tests confirm damage of vestibular function. Vestibular damage is seldom severe, and usually clears up after the drug is discontinued. Some patients develop tinnitus, and less commonly there is hearing loss; rarely this may progress to total deafness. Even more rarely, deafness may occur suddenly, without any warning whatsoever. Hearing loss of some extent occurs in many patients, but it is usually limited to the high frequency range and goes unnoticed by the patient, being detectable only by audiometric examination.

Renal toxicity is common but seldom severe; it is manifested by the presence of albumin and casts in the urine, but rarely is there damage to renal function. Albuminuria and cylindruria do not require cessation of viomycin therapy, and they usually disappear when the drug is stopped. However, viomycin should be given cautiously and in reduced dosage to those patients who already have damaged renal function, since these patients may develop high and toxic levels as a result of impaired excretion. Allergic manifestations are also fairly common, but seldom severe enough to require interruption of treatment. They take the form of drug fever, pruritus, maculopapular skin rashes, urticaria, localized edema and eosinophilia. The skin rashes often appear soon after the injection of viomycin and respond promptly to adrenalin or antihistamines. Reduction of serum electrolytes is not uncommon, potassium, calcium, and chlorides being lowered, and electrocardiographic changes developing which are consistent with hypokalemia. Lowered serum electrolytes may be treated adequately simply by the administration of potassium chloride (41).

Initially, most strains of tubercle bacilli are susceptible to viomycin, but a few strains exhibit primary resistance to this drug (42). Following treatment, resistance to viomycin develops as in the case of streptomycin, but at a slower rate (43). When the tubercle bacilli become resistant to 10 μg viomycin per ml, the drug is no longer helpful in treatment (41).

Summary

Viomycin is an antibiotic which is less effective in the treatment of tuberculosis than streptomycin or isoniazid but is nevertheless a valuable drug. Its toxic manifestations — renal irritation, allergic reactions, reduction of serum electrolytes, and impairment of the function of the eighth cranial nerve — are seldom severe enough to require abandonment of treatment with this drug. Because of its toxicity, it should not be used in the initial treatment of tuberculosis. But when treatment is needed, and when streptomycin, isoniazid and PAS cannot be used effectively because of drug resistance or toxicity, viomycin with a companion drug may be most helpful.

KANAMYCIN

Kanamycin is an antibiotic isolated by Umezawa and his associates in 1957 from Streptomyces kanamyceticus (44). It is somewhat similar to neomycin and streptomycin in chemical structure. Kanamycin sulfate is a white crystalline powder freely soluble in water, and is stable in aqueous solution over a p^H range of 2 to 11. It is poorly absorbed from the gastrointestinal tract, so that oral administration is not practical. After intramuscular injection it is rapidly absorbed, and reaches a peak level in the blood stream in about an hour. About two hours after injection the serum level begins to decline rapidly, and by the twelfth hour the level is very low and ineffective. If the drug is given in doses of 0.5 gm intramuscularly, twice daily, there is no accumulation in the blood stream.

Lower doses yield blood levels which cannot be relied upon to be effective, and indeed the Japanese studies indicate that total dosage of less than 4 gm weekly is seldom adequate. Kanamycin diffuses into the pleural and ascitic fluids and into the bile, but not into the spinal fluid. Excretion is entirely by way of the kidneys, and is rapid and fairly complete. Nearly 100 per cent of the injected drug is excreted unchanged in the urine in twenty-four hours.

Kanamycin has been shown to be effective in the test tube against a variety of bacteria, including Staphylococci, Salmonella, Shigella, and many coliform bacilli, as well as against tubercle bacilli.

In the treatment of tuberculosis, the recommended dose of kanamycin is 0.5 gm intramuscularly, twice daily. In this dosage the drug is not highly effective. Sputum conversion is rare, fever comes down much more slowly than on streptomycin or isoniazid therapy, and x-ray clearing is slow and incomplete. Still, the drug usually causes some improvement, and progression of tuberculosis while on kanamycin therapy is uncommon. Kanamycin is active against tubercle bacilli which are resistant to streptomycin, isoniazid, cycloserine, and PAS, but is not active against bacilli which are resistant to neomycin or viomycin.

The factor which limits the use of kanamycin is its toxicity, particularly its toxicity for the auditory branch of the eighth nerve. The majority of patients who receive this drug for a prolonged period of time develop some measure of hearing loss, and it usually appears before the sixtieth day of treatment (45). Hearing loss for the upper frequencies is affected first, and this is often accompanied by tinnitus. Hearing loss is usually bilateral. It is related to the duration of treatment and to the serum level of the drug. When hearing loss manifests itself, kanamycin should be stopped at once. The damage to hearing is not reversible, but if the drug is stopped it usually does not progress; however, if administration of the drug is continued, hearing loss is likely to progress until total deafness exists. Indeed, cases are known where partial hearing loss due to kanamycin progressed to total deafness even after the drug was stopped. The risk of ototoxicity is least in young people with normal kidney function. When kanamycin is given for a long time, audiometric examinations should be done frequently, and if evidence of hearing loss develops, the drug should be stopped at once. Vestibular damage is much less common than hearing loss, but it does occur.

Because it is closely related to neomycin chemically, and because neomycin can produce severe nephrotoxicity, the toxicity of kanamycin for the kidney has been investigated thoroughly. It has been found that renal toxicity is not severe (46). Mild renal irritation, as evidenced by casts and sometimes by albuminuria and microscopic hematuria, is quite common but is reversible and does not require discontinuation of the drug unless there is damage to kidney function. Evidence of damage to renal function, such as a rising nonprotein nitrogen or blood urea nitrogen or a diminished PSP retention, is quite uncommon but does occur sometimes, and there has even been a case report of acute tubular necrosis. Kanamycin has been used in the treatment of renal tuberculosis, and even here, significant damage to renal function is uncommon. It is rarely necessary to discontinue kanamycin because of renal toxicity.

Other toxic manifestations are unimportant. Irritation or pain at the site of injection is often complained of, but is seldom severe enough to require discontinuation of treatment. Other side effects are rare, but include skin rash, abdominal discomfort, nausea, vomiting, diarrhoea, headache and paresthesias. Drug allergy is rare, but when it occurs, the drug must be stopped or desensitization carried out.

Tubercle bacilli which are already resistant to neomycin or viomycin are likely to be resistant to kanamycin from the start. Otherwise there is little or no primary resistance to kanamycin. Tubercle bacilli develop resistance to kanamycin very rapidly when exposed to this drug alone, a high degree of resistance (to 1000 μg per ml) occurring after only four transfers in the test tube. However, the use of a second drug in combination with kanamycin greatly delays the development of resistance. The resistant organisms are fully virulent for experimental animals and probably for man (47).

Summary

Kanamycin is moderately effective against tubercle bacilli when used in doses of 0.5 gm twice daily, intramuscularly. In these doses, however, it produces serious hearing loss in the great majority of patients (48), the loss being apparent between the thirtieth and the sixtieth day of treatment in most cases. If treatment is continued after hearing loss manifests itself, it is likely to progress to total deafness. Smaller doses are less toxic but are also less effective. Because of its ototoxicity, kanamycin is not widely used. It may be used for long periods in doses of 0.5 gm twice daily, three or four days weekly, but its effectiveness in these doses is limited. Kanamycin finds its greatest usefulness when a drug is needed for a relatively brief period (as when resectional surgery is necessary) and when the tubercle bacilli are resistant to other drugs.

THIOCARBANIDIN

Thiocarbanidin is a phenylthiourea derivative prepared by Doub and his associates and found by them to have antituberculosis activity (49). It is only slightly soluble in water. When given by mouth in doses of 1 gm daily, peak serum levels of 0.2 μg to 1.7 μg, with an average of 0.9 μg, are reached in two to four hours. In rats, the concentration in many tissues is much higher than in the blood. Much the highest drug concentrations are reached in body fat depots, fully ten times as high as in the serum. High concentrations are also found in the liver, and lower but significant concentrations in the heart, kidney, lung and spleen (50). Thiocarbanidin persists in the blood and tissues for several days. Detectable quantities exist in the blood for two days after the last dose, and the drug is found even longer in the urine. Thiocarbanidin is absorbed poorly from the gastrointestinal tract, about 95 per cent of the total amount ingested appearing in the feces in man. That portion which is absorbed is excreted slowly in the urine, but only 0.14 to 0.31 per cent of the total ingested drug can be recovered from the urine (51). In spite of the high tissue concentration in the liver, none of the drug is excreted in the bile.

Thiocarbanidin has been shown to be effective against tubercle bacilli in the test tube, concentrations of 0.5 μg per ml inhibiting tubercle bacilli, even those which are resistant to isoniazid and PAS (52). In mice infected with tuberculosis, the drug definitely prolongs the survival time. It is far inferior to streptomycin and isoniazid, and it is even inferior to PAS in effectiveness. The drug is unusual in this respect, that large increases in its dose do not cause proportional increase in its antituberculosis activity (49). By itself, thiocarbanidin has proved to be a feebly active drug in animal tuberculosis. Used with isoniazid, thiocarbanidin is inferior to PAS in therapeutic efficacy in the treatment of tuberculosis in monkeys. In human tuberculosis, when used in doses of 2 gm per day with streptomycin or isoniazid, thiocarbanidin does not prevent the development of resistance to these drugs as well as PAS does, nor is it as useful in reversing infectiousness or in preventing the spread of disease (53) (54).

Thiocarbanidin does not cause any serious toxicity. It sometimes causes drug fever, leukopenia, skin rashes or gastrointestinal complaints, but these have only occasionally required that the drug be stopped, and have never been serious (54). Both the lack of effectiveness and toxicity of this drug are probably due to poor absorption from the gastrointestinal tract of man (50) (55).

Primary resistance to thiocarbanidin has not been reported. However, whenever the sputum remains positive after four months of combined therapy including this drug, resistance to thiocarbanidin has developed in almost all cases and resistance to the companion drug has developed in about 75 per cent of cases.

Summary

Thiocarbanidin is a thiourea derivative which is feebly active against tubercle bacilli in the test tube and in mice. It is relatively nontoxic. Because it is poorly absorbed from the gastrointestinal tract in man, it is almost ineffective in the treatment of clinical tuberculosis. Its only possible usefulness is as a substitute for PAS in cases in which PAS is poorly tolerated.

THE THIOSEMICARBAZONES

Interest in the possible value of the complex sulfur-containing compounds in the treatment of tuberculosis was aroused in the middle 1940's. Many such compounds were synthesized and tested in Germany as early as 1946, and the thiosemicarbazones were found to be the most effective of them all. The most widely used of the thiosemicarbazones was amithiozone (Conteban, Tibione, or Tb-1). Other related compounds were also found to be effective, but the compounds which were more bacteriostatic were also more toxic, and were therefore soon given up.

Amithiozone is given orally. It is absorbed satisfactorily from the gastrointestinal tract and appears in the serum in maximum concentrations about four hours after an oral dose is ingested. Following a dose of 400 mg a serum level of about 1 μg per ml is achieved. It rapidly diffuses into the various organs, reaching different concentrations in different organs. A concentration of 3 μg per gram is readily reached in the lungs, and this is bacteriostatic. Amithiozone passes the placental barrier, and reaches the fetal circulation in significant concentration. The drug is excreted slowly by the kidneys, about 40 per cent appearing in the urine in the first forty-eight hours. It is also excreted in the milk. Since much of it remains in the tissues for several days, it tends to accumulate if administered daily.

Amithiozone is administered by mouth. Because of toxicity, it is customary to start treatment with small doses, and to increase to 100 mg daily (in divided doses) by a series of steps. In concentrations of 1 μg per ml amithiozone inhibits the growth of tubercle bacilli in the test tube. In experimental tuberculosis, too, this drug is an effective tuberculostatic. These promising results cannot, however, be duplicated in clinical tuberculosis. It is true that its use results in improvement in laryngeal, bronchial and intestinal tuberculosis and in exudative pulmonary tuberculosis, but in other forms of tuberculosis it is usually without value (56) (57). On the whole, amithiozone is rather a feeble antituberculosis drug.

It is possible that in larger doses amithiozone would be more effective. Large doses are well tolerated by mice, guinea pigs and other experimental animals, but in man large doses are toxic. The largest dose which is tolerated by man is about 5 mg per kg, and even this results in many toxic manifestations. The dose which has been accepted is 100 mg daily, in divided doses, and even this small amount produces considerable toxicity (58). Toxicity, when it occurs, usually manifests itself during the first three months of treatment. Anorexia, nausea and vomiting are the commonest evidences of toxicity. The most serious forms of toxicity are those involving the hematopoietic system—progressive anemia is not uncommon, and granulocytopenia and even a few cases of agranulocytosis have been reported.

Liver damage is not common but many may be serious and may occur at any time during treatment; this is demonstrated by bromsulfalein retention and occasionally by jaundice. Renal impairment is also seen occasionally, and manifests itself by a rising blood urea nitrogen and by the presence of albumin and red blood cells in the urine. Drug fever and skin rashes are also seen occasionally. Most of these adverse effects are transient and disappear promptly when the drug is discontinued, but sometimes agranulocytosis, liver damage or kidney damage may be serious or even fatal. All in all, a very high percentage of patients who receive amithiozone suffer from the drug's toxicity, and sometimes this toxicity is serious.

Initial resistance to amithiozone sometimes exists, without any previous exposure to this drug, but this is not common. When amithiozone is given alone, resistance develops rapidly. When it is given with streptomycin, it does not delay the development of resistance to streptomycin much; it is not nearly as effective as PAS in this regard. Tubercle bacilli which are resistant to amithiozone remain fully virulent.

It can be seen from the above discussion that amithiozone is a drug of limited effectiveness and considerable toxicity. It does not have the virtue of delaying the development of resistance to the major drugs when it is used in conjunction with them. It is, in fact, a third rate drug which is now of historical interest only. Actually, amithiozone is no longer on the market.

Amithiozone, however, feeble and toxic though it is, does have some effect against tubercle bacilli in the test tube and in experimental animals, and is of some value in tuberculosis of the mucous membranes in man. Though it has been abandoned, many other thiosemicarbazones have been investigated in the test tube and in experimental tuberculosis, and several have been promising enough to deserve study in clinical tuberculosis. The most recently studied of these compounds is isoxyl.

Isoxyl has been administered to experimental animals both by mouth and intravenously. The oral drug has produced no toxic manifestations, but when the drug has been used intravenously it has produced hypotension and even cardiac arrest. This drug is poorly absorbed from the gastrointestinal tract, and the small amount which reaches the blood stream is, in large part, bound to the plasma proteins. It is possible that the low toxicity of this drug when given orally is due to the very small amount which reaches the blood and tissues. Isoxyl shows little activity against experimental tuberculosis in monkeys, probably due to its poor absorption from the gastrointestinal tract (59). Studies of the effect of isoxyl in human tuberculosis have thus far not shown impressive results, but controlled clinical trials are still being carried out.

Summary

Drugs of the thiosemicarbazone series have been used intermittently for almost twenty years. Of them all, amithiozone received the widest clinical trial. It proved to be feebly active, rather toxic, and not even helpful as a companion drug, since it did not significantly delay the development of resistance to the primary drug. It has therefore been abandoned. The search for better drugs of the same general class has continued until the present time. Although no valuable drug has yet emerged as a direct result of this search, it was as an intermediary product in the synthesis of a thiosemicarbazone that attention was first drawn to the best of the antituberculosis drugs, isoniazid.

REFERENCES

1. GRUMBACH, F., RIST, N., LIBERMANN, D., MOYEUX, M., CALS, S., AND CLAVEL, S.: Antitubercular activity of some isonicotinic thioamides with substitutions on the nucleus. *C. R. Acad. Sci.,* *242*:2187, 1956.

2. GREENBERG, L., AND EIDUS, L.: Antituberculous drugs (TH 1314 and INH) in the host organism. *Brit. J. Dis. Chest, 56*:124, 1962.

3. EULE, H., AND WERNER, E.: Serum and urine levels of ethionamide. *Tuberkulosearzt, 15*:806, 1961.

4. HUGHES, I. E., SMITH, H., AND KANE, P. O.: Ethionamide: Its passage into the cerebrospinal fluid in man. *Lancet, 1*:616, 1962.
5. GRAY, D. G., HAMILTON, E. J., AND EIDUS, L.: Clinical-laboratory studies of Alpha-ethyl-thioisonicatinamide (TH 1314). *Canad. Med. Ass. J., 86*:317, 1962.
6. YAMAMOTO, M., YAMAGUCHI, W., KUMAZAWA, Y., AND TAKAHASHI, Y.: The fate of ethionamide *in vivo. Jap. J. Chest Dis., 6*:1036, 1962.
7. BROUET, G., MARCHE, J., RIST, N., CHEVALLIER, J., AND LE MEUR, G.: Studies on the antitubercular activity of alpha-ethyl-thioisonicotinamide in human tuberculosis. *Amer. Rev. Tuberc., 79*:6, 1959.
8. SCHWARTZ, W. S.: A comparison of ethionamide with isoniazid in original treatment cases. *Trans. 23rd Research Conference Pulmonary Diseases*, p. 13, 1964.
9. MATTHEWS, J. H.: Thioamide in various combinations in retreatment pulmonary tuberculosis. *Trans. 20th Research Conference Pulmonary Diseases*, p. 146, 1961.
10. LEES, A. W.: Toxicity in newly diagnosed cases of pulmonary tuberculosis treated with ethionamide. *Amer. Rev. Resp. Dis., 88*:347, 1963.
11. LEGGAT, P. O.: Ethionamide neuropathy. *Tubercle, 43*:95, 1962.
12. MOULDING, T. S., JR., AND GOLDSTEIN, S.: Hepatoxicity due to ethionamide. *Amer. Rev. Resp. Dis., 86*:252, 1962.
13. PHILLIPS, S., AND TASHMAN, H.: Ethionamide jaundice. *Amer. Rev. Resp. Dis., 87*:896, 1963.
14. McCUNE, R., AND TOMPSETT, R.: Effect of pyrazinamide—isoniazid and other antituberculous drugs on populations of M. tuberculosis in experimental animals. *Trans. Thirteenth Conference Chemotherapy Tuberculosis*, p. 168, 1954.
15. PHILLIPS, S., AND HORTON, G. E.: Pyrazinamide-isoniazid. Companion with isoniazid—PAS in active pulmonary tuberculosis. *Amer. Rev. Tuberc., 73*:704, 1956.
16. McDERMOTT, W., ORMOND, L., MUSCHENHEIM, C., DEUSCHLE, K., McCUNE, R. M., AND TOMPSETT, R.: Pyrazinamide—isoniazid in tuberculosis. *Amer. Rev. Tuberc., 69*:319, 1954.
17. SPENGOS, T. N., AND CUIZON, R.: Pyrazinamide-induced acute yellow atrophy of the liver. *Amer. Rev. Tuberc., 77*:858, 1958.
18. CULLEN, J. H., EARLY, J. A. E., AND FIORE, J. M.: The occurrence of hyperuricemia during pyrazinamide-isoniazid therapy. *Amer. Rev. Tuberc., 74*:280, 1956.

19. MODAVE, J.: Cycloserine and its value in the treatment of chronic pulmonary tuberculosis. *Antibiot. Med. Clin. Ther., 4*:535, 1957.
20. RENZETTI, A. D., WRIGHT, K. W., EDLING, J. H., AND BUNN, P.: Clinical bacteriologic, and pharmacologic observations upon cycloserine. *Amer. Rev. Tuberc., 74*:128, 1956.
21. CONZELMAN, G. M.: The physiologic disposition of cycloserine in the human subject. *Amer. Rev. Tuberc., 74*:739, 1956.
22. CUMMINGS, M. M., PATNODE, R. A., AND HUDGINS, P. C.: Effects of cycloserine on M. tuberculosis *in vitro, Trans. 14th Conference Chemotherapy Tuberculosis,* p. 321, 1955.
23. STEENKEN, W., AND WOLINSKY, E.: Cycloserine: antituberculous activity *in vitro* and in the experimental animal. *Amer. Rev. Tuberc., 73*:539, 1956.
24. EPSTEIN, I. G., NAIR, K. G. S., AND BOYD, L. J.: Cycloserine in the treatment of human pulmonary tuberculosis. *Trans. 14th Conference Chemotherapy Tuberculosis,* p. 326, 1955.
25. COHEN, A. C., AND DROSS, I. C.: High-dosage cycloserine in treatment failures. *Trans. 19th Conference Chemotherapy Tuberculosis,* p. 173, 1960.
26. LEVI-VALENSI, A., POROT, M., LEONARDON, P., DALET, R., AND MIGUERES, J.: Les accidents neuropsychiatriques survenant chez les tuberculeux traites par la cycloserine. *Ann. Med. Psychol., 115*:899, 1957.
27. VIALLIER, J., AND CAYRE, R. M.: Bacilles tuberculeux resistants a la cycloserine. *C. R. Soc. Biol., 152*:776, 1958.
28. KARLSON, A. G.: The *in vitro* activity of ethambutol (dextro-2,2' ((ethylenediimino))-d-1-butanol) against tubercle bacilli and other microorganisms. *Amer. Rev. Resp. Dis., 84*:905, 1961.
29. ROBINSON, L. B., AND WICHELHAUSEN, R.: *In vitro* studies on two recently developed antituberculous agents: ethambutol and capreomycin. *Trans. 21st Research Conference Pulmonary Diseases,* p. 351, 1962.
30. PLACE, V. A., AND THOMAS, J. P.: Clinical pharmacology of ethambutol. *Amer. Rev. Resp. Dis., 87*:901, 1963.
31. PEETS, E. A., AND BUYAKE, D. A.: Studies of the metabolism in the dog of ethambutol—C14, a drug having antituberculosis activity. *Pharmacologist, 4*:171, 1962.
32. SCHMIDT, L. H., GOOD, R. C., MACK, H. P., ZEEK-MINNING, P., AND SCHMIDT, I. G.: An experimental appraisal of the therapeutic potentialities of ethambutol. *Trans. 22nd Research Conference Pulmonary Diseases,* p. 262, 1963.

33. BOBROWITZ, I. D., GARBER, M., AND SUKUMALCHANTRE, Y.: The use of ethambutol in pulmonary tuberculosis. *Trans. 22nd Research Conference Pulmonary Diseases*, p. 254, 1963.
34. BOBROWITZ, I. D., AND GOKULANATHAN, K. S.: Ethambutol in the retreatment of pulmonary tuberculosis. *Dis. Chest, 48*:239, 1965.
35. HERR, E. B., SUTTON, W. B., AND STARK, W. M.: Chemical and biological studies of capreomycin. *Trans. 21st Research Conference Pulmonary Diseases*, p. 367, 1962.
36. MILLER, J. D., LANDWEHR, A., GREENE, M. E., AND POPPLEWELL, A. G.: Effect of capreomycin in humans with pulmonary tuberculosis. *Trans. 21st Research Conference Pulmonary Diseases*, p. 370, 1962.
37. POPPLEWELL, A. G., MILLER, J. D., LANDWEHR, A., AND GREENE, M. E.: Capreomycin used in original treatment of advanced pulmonary tuberculosis. *Trans. 22nd Research Conference Pulmonary Diseases*, p. 275, 1963.
38. WERNER, C. A., ADAMS, C., AND DuBOIS, R.: Absorption and excretion of viomycin in humans. *Proc. Soc. Exp. Biol., 76*:292, 1951.
39. STEENKEN, W., AND WOLINSKY, E.: Viomycin in experimental tuberculosis. *Amer. Rev. Tuberc., 63*:30, 1951.
40. YOUMANS, G. P., AND YOUMANS, A. S.: The effect of viomycin *in vitro* and *in vivo* on M. tuberculosis. *Amer. Rev. Tuberc., 63*:25, 1951.
41. TUCKER, W. B.: Retreatment of advanced pulmonary tuberculosis with viomycin. *Amer. Rev. Tuberc., 70*:812, 1954.
42. VALLIER, J., AND CAYRE, R. M.: Sur la sensibilite a la viomycine de 189 souches de M. tuberculosis. *C. R. Soc. Biol., 151*:1925, 1958.
43. HOBBY, G.: Viomycin: Summary of a four-year evaluation. *Trans. Twelfth Conference Chemotherapy Tuberculosis*, p. 300, 1953.
44. UMEZAWA, H.: Kanamycin: Its discovery. *Ann. N. Y. Acad. Sci., 76*:20, 1958.
45. HAWKINS, J. E., FROST, J. O., AND DALY, J. F.: The ototoxicity of kanamycin in tuberculous patients. *Trans. 18th Conference Chemotherapy Tuberculosis*, p. 339, 1959.
46. BERMAN, L. B., AND KATZ, S.: Kanamycin nephrotoxicity. *Ann. N. Y. Acad. Sci., 76*:149, 1958.
47. STEENKEN, W., MONTALBINE, V., AND THURSTON, J. R.: The antituberculous activity of kanamycin *in vitro* and in the experimental animal. *Trans. 17th Conference Chemotherapy Tuberculosis*, p. 386, 1958.

48. SCHWARTZ, W. S.: Kanamycin in the treatment of pulmonary tuberculosis. *Trans. 18th Conference Chemotherapy Tuberculosis,* p. 343, 1959.

49. YOUMANS, G. P., YOUMANS, A. S., AND DOUB, L.: The effect of thiocarbanidin on mycobacterium tuberculosis *in vitro* and *in vivo. Trans. 17th Conference Chemotherapy Tuberculosis,* p. 365, 1958.

50. DILL, W. A., AND GLAZKO, A. J.: Metabolism of Y-9525 (Thiocarbanidin). *Trans. 17th Conference Chemotherapy Tuberculosis,* p. 373, 1958.

51. SCHMIDT, L. H., GROVER, A. A., AND HOFFMAN, R.: The comparative therapeutic activities of thiocarbanidin and para-aminosalicylic acid administered alone and in combination with isoniazid. *Trans. 18th Conference Chemotherapy Tuberculosis,* p. 312, 1959.

52. STEENKEN, W., MONTALBINE, V., SMITH, M. M., AND WOLINSKY, E.: Antituberculous activity of thiocarbanidin *in vitro* and in the experimental animal. *Trans. 17th Conference Chemotherapy Tuberculosis,* p. 368, 1958.

53. DONOHOE, R. F., KATZ, S., DUKE, C. J., AND ROMANSKY, M. J.: An evaluation of thiocarbanidin and isonicotinic acid hydrazide in the treatment of pulmonary tuberculosis. *Trans. 18th Conference Chemotherapy Tuberculosis,* p. 317, 1959.

54. LARKIN, J. C.: Results of therapy with thiocarbanidin used with isoniazid or streptomycin. *Amer. Rev. Resp. Dis., 81*:235, 1960.

55. GRUMBACH, F., AND RIST, N.: Comparison de l' activité antituberculeuse experimentale de la thiocarbanidine et de l' ethionamide. *Ann. Inst. Pasteur (Paris), 98*:373, 1960.

56. HINSHAW, H. C., AND McDERMOTT, W.: Thiosemicarbasone therapy of tuberculosis in humans. *Amer. Rev. Tuberc., 61*:145, 1950.

57. SANDHAUS, H. S., JENKINS, D. E., BURDON, K. L., AND HALPERT, B., Amithiozone treatment of pulmonary tuberculosis. *Amer. Rev. Tuberc., 64*:170, 1951.

58. SKAVLEM, J. H., HUMPHREY, H. I., WOLIUNG, R. W., AND SPRINKLE, R. P.: Thiosemicarbasones in tuberculosis. *Trans. Tenth Conference Chemotherapy Tuberculosis,* p. 120, 1951.

59. GOOD, R. C., HOFFMANN, R. A., SMITH, C. C., AND SCHMIDT, L.: Observations on the prophylactic and therapeutic properties of isoxyl. *Trans. Twenty-third Research Conference Pulmonary Diseases,* p. 10, 1964.

Chapter VI

ADRENOCORTICOSTEROID HORMONES

THE ADRENOCORTICOSTEROID hormones have many actions. As far as tuberculosis is concerned, some of their effects are harmful and some may be helpful. These steroids impair the ability of macrophages to engulf and destroy tubercle bacilli, and they interfere with the production of lymphocytes and with antibody formation (1). By these and other mechanisms they lower the resistance of the host to tubercle bacilli. Much more important is their anti-inflammatory action, which may be disastrous, but which may in some circumstances be turned to advantage.

The first experience with these hormones in tuberculosis was catastrophic. Because of their anti-inflammatory action they were widely used in the management of arthritis, and they were used for long periods of time. This lowered the host resistance to tuberculosis, handicapping several of the mechanisms of resistance, and resulted in progression of disease in many cases of active tuberculosis, and in the reactivation of many inactive tuberculous lesions. It is true that many times adrenocorticosteroids were administered to patients with inactive tuberculosis without causing flare-ups, but so frequent were reports of exacerbation in these circumstances that the use of these steroids in active or even inactive tuberculosis came to be regarded as dangerous.

The steroids have no effect on the growth and multiplication of tubercle bacilli in the test tube. In experimental tuberculosis the steroid hormones have generally a deleterious effect, causing the disease to progress more rapidly. They do this by lowering the resistance of the infected animal, and especially by reducing or abolishing the inflammatory reaction which tends to surround and localize the infectious process. Both in animals (2), and in human beings it has been found that this deleterious effect of the steroids can be counteracted by the simultaneous use of antituberculosis drugs.

When effective antituberculosis drugs are used at the same time, it is safe to administer the corticosteroids. The first lesson to be learned from these facts is this: When it is desirable to give prolonged steroid therapy, for any reason, to a patient who has a tuberculous infection, effective antituberculosis drugs should be administered at the same time. This is true whether the tuberculous infection takes the form of active tuberculosis, inactive tuberculosis, or even a positive tuberculin reaction alone. But the anti-inflammatory action of the steroids is not entirely disadvantageous. Since their harmful effects can be counteracted by effective antituberculosis drugs, they may be used for their possible beneficial effects. On theoretical grounds it has been proposed that the use of steroid hormones, always accompanied by effective antituberculosis drugs to prevent dissemination of disease, might reduce inflammation and thereby reduce tissue destruction, so that later scar tissue formation and resulting damage to pulmonary function would be minimized.

It has also been supposed that by the reduction of inflammation the steroids would favor the more rapid clearing of exudative tuberculous lesions. Neither of these suppositions has been proved to happen. There is as yet no proof of the tissue-sparing effect of the steroids. As far as more rapid clearing is concerned, it is true that patients with acute exudative tuberculosis who are treated with steroids as well as effective antituberculosis drugs do have a more rapid reduction of fever, and their lesions clear more rapidly in the first month or two; however, after six months of treatment they have made no more progress than their fellow patients who have received the same antituberculosis drugs without steroids.

There are several situations in which the adrenocorticosteroid drugs have found a limited field of usefulness as an adjunct to chemotherapy in the treatment of tuberculosis (3) (4) (5).

1. *Fulminating, rapidly progressive pulmonary tuberculosis* may result in death in a few weeks. Here the steroids may arrest the downhill course long enough to tip the balance in the direction of recovery, providing time for the antituberculosis drugs to become effective. The dose of 20-25 mg of prednisolone or its equivalent is given three times daily at first, and this is gradually reduced, titrating the dose against the patient's symptoms and endeavoring to keep him

free of fever. A maintenance dose of 5 to 10 mg of prednisolone or its equivalent should be continued for two or three weeks, and then the drug may be tapered off. The symptomatic improvement is likely to be dramatic, and in some cases the addition of steroids to the therapy may be lifesaving. There are bound to be many failures of course; steroids cannot be counted on to salvage a high percentage of patients who are in an advanced stage of malnutrition as a result of overwhelming tuberculous disease (5).

2. *In miliary tuberculosis* the same regimen may be extremely helpful. The use of steroids results in the miliary tubercles becoming smaller because of the absence or reduction of the zone of inflammation surrounding them. The numerous bacilli in these tubercles are inhibited by the standard antituberculosis drugs which must be administered at the same time.

3. *In tuberculous meningitis* the early use of adrenocorticosteroid drugs may be lifesaving (6). The regime should be the same, though the duration of treatment may have to be longer. Here the steroids favor the reduction of inflammation and the absorption of the exudate, and this is a great advantage.

4. *In large serous pleural and pericardial effusions,* steroids favor the absorption of the fluid and minimize the formation of adhesions.

5. *Tuberculous lymphadenitis* may resolve more rapidly when the standard therapy is bolstered for the first few weeks by steroids.

6. *Hypersensitivity reactions* to antituberculosis drugs may be neutralized by steroids, permitting a useful drug to be continued.

In these circumstances the corticosteroid drugs may not only shorten the course of the disease but may, in some cases, actually reverse the otherwise fatal progression of the disease.

It cannot be said too often that the *adrenocorticosteroids* reduce inflammation and depress host resistance to tuberculosis. They *must, therefore, never be used in tuberculous patients without the simultaneous use of antituberculosis drugs,* and the knowledge that the tubercle bacilli involved are susceptible to those drugs. If the patient has had no previous treatment with the antituberculosis drugs, it is reasonably safe to use the steroids along with any two of the major antituberculosis drugs. If the patient has had previous chemotherapy, the use of the steroids requires the concomitant use of two drugs not previously used, or the use of two drugs proven by laboratory examination to be effective against the tubercle bacilli excreted by the patient.

Summary

The adrenocorticosteroid hormones, used alone, have a deleterious effect on the tuberculous patient. By suppressing the inflammatory reaction to infection, and by a variety of other mechanisms, they lower the resistance of the patient to tubercle bacilli and favor progression of the disease. When they are to be used for the treatment of other disease in a patient infected with tuberculosis, it is imperative that antituberculosis drugs be administered at the same time. The steroids must not be used in the tuberculous patient unless the tubercle bacilli are susceptible to the major drugs. There are a few special situations in which the steroid hormones, always accompanied by effective antituberculosis drugs, may be used to advantage in the treatment of tuberculosis. These are fulminating pulmonary tuberculosis, miliary and meningeal tuberculosis, massive pleural and pericardial effusions, and some cases of tuberculous lymphadenitis and of hypersensitivity to antituberculosis drugs.

Under chemotherapeutic protection these hormones can be used with a considerable degree of safety. It is not recommended that they should be used often, but in the special circumstances mentioned above their use should be considered. Occasionally the steroids may be lifesaving.

REFERENCES

1. LURIE, M. B., ZAPPASODI, P., AND TICKNER, C.: On the nature of genetic resistance to tuberculosis in the light of the host-parasite relationships in natively resistant and susceptible rabbits. *Amer. Rev. Tuberc.*, 72:297, 1955.
2. BACOS, J. M., AND SMITH, D. T.: The effect of corticotropin (ACTH), dihydrostreptomycin ,and corticotropin-dihydrostreptomycin on experimental bovine tuberculosis in the rabbit. *Amer. Rev. Tuberc.*, 67:201, 1953.
3. HORNE, N. W.: Prednisolone in treatment of pulmonary tuberculosis. *Brit. Med. J.*, 2:1751, 1960.

4. Committee on Therapy, American Trudeau Society, Drug treatment of pulmonary tuberculosis. *Amer. Rev. Resp. Dis., 81*:438, 1960.
5. JOHNSON, J. R., TAYLOR, B. C., MORRISSEY, J. F., JENNE, J. W., AND MacDONALD, F. M.: Corticosteroids in pulmonary tuberculosis. *Am. Rev. Resp. Dis., 92*:376, 1965.
6. SIMPSON, D. G., AND McCLEMENT, J. H.: Adrenal corticosteroids in life-threatening pulmonary tuberculosis. *Amer. Rev. Resp. Dis., 90*:754, 1964.
7. COCCHI, C.: Cortisone and corticotropin in the treatment of tuberculosis in childhood. *Amer. Rev. Tuberc., 74*:209, 1956.

Chapter VII

INITIAL TREATMENT OF CHRONIC PULMONARY TUBERCULOSIS

A NUMBER OF PRINCIPLES should guide us in the management of a new case of chronic pulmonary tuberculosis. Some of the principles are as follows:

1. The first course of treatment should be adequate in every way. Never again will there be as good an opportunity to cure the disease.
2. Drug treatment is the basis of all successful treatment of pulmonary tuberculosis. Rest, surgery and other forms of therapy may sometimes be used, but if they are needed they are adjuncts to drug treatment.
3. Two drugs should be used.
4. Two effective drugs should be used. The choice of drugs should be guided by drug-susceptibility tests.
5. Treatment should be prolonged.
6. Treatment should be uninterrupted.
7. The drugs should be changed if change is indicated.

It seems self-evident that the first course of treatment should be fully effective, but often the first course is deficient in some respect. At least 10 per cent of treated patients fail to recover, and in most cases failure is due to inadequacy of treatment. Too often, for instance, the physician discontinues PAS because the patient suffers from mild nausea and anorexia, or the patient stops taking this drug because of minor symptoms, not understanding the importance of taking his treatment faithfully. Too often the patient takes his drugs irregularly or discontinues them altogether because he becomes discouraged with the slowness of his progress. Too often the patient takes his drugs irregularly or discontinues them altogether for the opposite reason—because all his symptoms have disappeared, his appetite has returned, he has regained the weight lost, and he believes that he is well and needs no more treatment.

In the great majority of cases, treatment failure is due to inadequacy of treatment in some respect. The commonest error of treatment is the failure to take the drugs faithfully, without interruption, for a long time. Failure to produce inactivity of pulmonary tuberculosis with the first course of treatment is unfortunate, because a second course is not likely to be as effective as the first. The patient may have become hypersensitive to one drug or another, or the tubercle bacilli may have developed some degree of resistance to one drug or another as a result of the first course of treatment, and these changes make retreatment less likely to be successful than initial treatment. It is most desirable to make the first course of treatment completely effective. Never again will the patient have as good an opportunity to make a complete and permanent recovery from tuberculosis.

Not only is the first course of treatment the most likely to be successful, but healing the disease as early as possible minimizes tissue damage and later scarring. If tissue injury is considerable, even if the patient recovers it may be at the cost of severe impairment of respiratory function. In such patients, comfort is reduced, health is damaged, and life itself may be shortened. This is an additional reason why the first course of treatment should be made as effective as possible.

Drug treatment is the foundation of all treatment of tuberculosis. All cases of active tuberculosis deserve treatment with the antituberculosis drugs, even the most minimal cases. All other forms of treatment are accessory. If surgery is desirable, it should be preceded and followed by drug therapy. Bed rest still has a limited role in the management of pulmonary tuberculosis, but it should not be relied upon for the therapy of even the most minimal cases without the addition of the antituberculosis drugs.

Ordinarily two drugs should be used for the treatment of pulmonary tuberculosis. Non-cavitary pulmonary tuberculosis has been treated successfully with isoniazid alone, but even in these cases two-drug therapy yields better results with regard to clinical and radiological improvement, sputum conversion, and the emergence of strains of tubercle bacilli resistant to isoniazid (1).

Not only is two-drug therapy more effective than therapy with a single drug, but the development of drug-resistant strains of tubercle bacilli is postponed and may usually be prevented altogether by the simultaneous use of two drugs. Some have urged that if two drugs are better than one, perhaps the use of three drugs simultaneously would be even better. Actually there is some evidence that this is so. In the case of genitourinary tuberculosis triple-drug therapy appears to be a little more effective than therapy with two drugs.

In life-threatening forms of the disease such as miliary and meningeal tuberculosis, therapy with three drugs is always recommended. In chronic pulmonary tuberculosis, evidence is beginning to accumulate indicating that three drugs are a little more effective than two. The difference is not great, however, and the addition of a third drug significantly increases the toxicity. A reasonable compromise may be the initial employment of three drugs for a limited period, perhaps six weeks, followed by a long period of two-drug therapy. In most cases two-drug therapy is entirely adequate, but the most important time in the treatment of tuberculosis is in the beginning, when the bacilli should be attacked by a battery of drugs which are entirely effective. Whether two drugs or three are used at the beginning, isoniazid should always be part of the initial treatment unless there is a contraindication.

The physician should assure himself that the drugs he is employing are fully effective, that is, the tubercle bacilli are susceptible to them. Treatment should be guided throughout by the results of drug-susceptibility testing. Many treatment failures are the consequence of employing drugs to which the bacilli are partially or entirely resistant. The methods used in testing susceptibility or resistance are well described in the *Handbook of Tuberculosis Laboratory Methods* (2). The first positive culture should be tested for drug-susceptibility, and thereafter monthly cultures should be rechecked as long as the sputum remains positive. If two drugs are used, and the bacilli are resistant to one but susceptible to the other, resistance to the second will develop quickly and the drug combination will no longer be useful.

While awaiting the results of drug-susceptibility tests, treatment should be started with drugs to which susceptibility is believed to exist (3).

The incidence of primary drug resistance in the United States is still low; in 1963 it was 1.9 per cent for streptomycin, 1.9 per cent for isoniazid, and 2.2 per cent for PAS (4). Any two-drug regimen is therefore likely to be effective, and any combination which includes isoniazid may be used. However, the original positive cultures should be checked for drug-susceptibility, and if resistance is found to exist to any drug (except isoniazid) which is being used, another drug should be substituted. In general, there is a fairly good correlation between drug-susceptibility as shown by laboratory tests and the clinical effectiveness of a drug.

Isoniazid is an exception to this rule; there is a good deal of evidence that the demonstration of resistance to isoniazid in the laboratory does not necessarily prove that the drug will not be clinically effective. Even when the bacilli are known to be isoniazid-resistant, good clinical responses are the rule when tuberculosis is treated with a combination of isoniazid and another drug (5). Therefore isoniazid may be continued, even when the bacilli are resistant to it, with the probability that it will be helpful. However, in this situation it should not be relied on as part of the two-drug combination, but should be used in addition. For instance, if treatment has been carried on successfully with isoniazid and PAS for two months and the laboratory reports that now the tubercle bacilli are resistant to isoniazed but are susceptible to streptomycin and PAS, a good combination would consist of three drugs, streptomycin, isoniazid and PAS.

Though a two-drug combination is usually perfectly effective, we have seen that there is some therapeutic advantage in starting treatment with three drugs. Another advantage of the initial use of three drugs is that, if there should be primary resistance to one drug, the patient will still receive the benefit of two effective drugs. The initial sputum should be cultured, of course, and the bacilli tested for drug susceptibility, and thereafter monthly sputum cultures should be done and tests for drug susceptibility should be carried out as long as cultures are positive. Treatment should always involve the use of two drugs of known effectiveness. If resistance develops to one of the drugs being used, but the organisms remain fully susceptible to the other, one new drug should be substituted. If complete resistance develops to one drug and partial resistance to the other, it is best to discard both drugs and to substitute two previously unused drugs of proven effectiveness.

Drug resistance seldom develops in children, or in adults with non-cavitary lesions. Good treatment requires the use of two drugs to which the bacilli are fully susceptible.

The duration of treatment should always be long. The theoretical reason for this is that the antituberculosis drugs act only on active, multiplying bacilli and not on resting bacilli, so that if these drugs are given for only a short time those tubercle bacilli which are in a resting state will not be affected; later these bacilli may grow, multiply and cause fresh disease. When the drugs are given for a longer period of time, resting tubercle bacilli which begin to grow are inhibited, so that long courses of treatment reduce the bacterial population much more than shorter courses. It has been established that relapses are far fewer when drugs have been given for a long time than when short courses of therapy have been employed.

How long treatment should be continued varies somewhat with the extent of the original lesion, and with the speed of sputum conversion, cavity closure and clearing by x-ray. Two years of chemotherapy is usually adequate, but this should be prolonged if the original lesion was very extensive, if sputum conversion was long delayed, if cavitation was slow to close, or if the clearing shown on successive x-rays was slow. In these situations, two-drug therapy should be continued for at least a year after sputum conversion and cavity closure have taken place and after the lesion has become stable by x-ray, and then therapy with isoniazid alone should be continued for another year or longer. When the original lesion was very large, or when cavities fail to close even though sputum conversion has occurred, treatment with isoniazid should be continued for a number of years or even indefinitely.

Interruption of treatment before the planned course has been completed is undesirable and may be disastrous. Not only is interrupted treatment far less effective than continuous treatment, but interruptions are likely to result in the early development of drug resistance, and treatment failure is a common consequence. Actually, repeated interruption of chemotherapy is probably the most frequent cause of treatment failure, so everything possible should be done to avoid it. Rarely, interruption is on the advice of a physician, who is so impressed by the speed of the resolution of exudative tuberculous lesions that he doubts the diagnosis and stops treatment. This is not common, surely, and yet it does happen sometimes when the diagnosis has been made without positive bacteriological proof. It should be a rule that if the evidence of tuberculosis is strong enough to justify beginning treatment a full course of treatment should be given.

Case Report

A white man, fifty-two years old, was well until March 1958, when he had fever, cough, weakness and loss of appetite. During the next month these symptoms persisted and he lost 12 pounds He entered a hospital on April 3, 1958. Temperature was 99.8°, examination showed rales over the lower half of the right chest, and x ray showed consolidation involving the right mid lung. Bronchoscopy was negative. Five sputum cultures were negative for acid-fast bacilli. Tuberculosis was suspected, and he was given streptomycin 1 gm daily, beginning April 16, 1958. The lesion cleared fairly rapidly, though incompletely. In the absence of bacteriological proof of tuberculosis, it was believed that the rapidity of the clearing ruled out tuberculosis, so streptomycin therapy was discontinued on June 25, 1958. He was seen again on July 29, 1958. There had been further resolution so he was discharged with the diagnosis of unresolved pneumonia. He had no further treatment for the pulmonary disease for six years.

In the summer of 1964, he developed the first of a series of "chest colds," with cough and expectoration. The cough became more severe and persistent, and there was weight loss, loss of appetite, and occasional fever. He was admitted to the hospital on February 24, 1965. Now x ray showed fluffy infiltration throughout the right lung, with a large cavity in the right apex and buckling of the trachea to the right. There was also some infiltration in the left upper lobe. Sputum was now consistently positive for acid-fast bacilli.

In retrospect, the lesion in the right middle lobe in 1958 was certainly tuberculous. A more determined effort would perhaps have identified tubercle bacilli in the secretions, but, although five sputum specimens were cultured for acid-fast bacilli and found negative, the sputum was scanty and neither bronchial secretions nor gastric washings were cultured. Once the tentative diagnosis of tuberculosis was made and chemotherapy started, this therapy should have been continued in the form of effective two-drug therapy. The lesion cleared rapidly but incompletely, and the unhealed lesion contained the seeds of the later spread of tuberculosis throughout the right lung and the left upper lobe. Continuous treatment would probably have cured this patient. Discontinuation of chemotherapy after ten weeks permitted the disease to smoulder and later to progress to far-advanced active cavitary tuberculosis.

Treatment is often interrupted when a patient leaves the hospital and goes home, or when he moves from one place to another. In this situation, it is the duty of the first physician to be sure that the physician or clinic which is going to be responsible for the future care of the patient is fully informed of the details of the patient's past treatment. It is a good practice to contact the new physician or clinic, give a resume of the case, and even make an appointment for the patient's first visit.

Most interruptions of treatment occur because the patient himself neglects to take his medication, usually for the most inconsequential reasons. Some reasons given are—"I had no more PAS, so took isoniazid alone." "I just don't like PAS," "The medicines cost too much," "It's too much trouble to go for my streptomycin shots," or, most often, "I felt good, and didn't think I needed the medicine any more." These reasons or excuses show that the patient often doesn't understand the importance of taking his medicine long and uninterruptedly to ensure healing and prevent relapses. In a recent interview, Fox has stated that the real reasons for difficulty in getting patients to take their medications at home for long periods are forgetfulness and indifference, since they feel perfectly well. Also some patients blame all their symptoms, no matter how unrelated, on their antituberculosis drugs (6).

Every effort should be made to impress on patients the vital necessity of taking their medication regularly. There will always be some treatment failures, but since the proper use of drugs can result in cure in almost 100 per cent of cases we should not tolerate treatment failures which result from negligence on the part of patients, poor communication between physicians and patients, or poor communications between physicians.

The persistence of cavitation is a serious matter. Untreated cavities are sources of infection, and from them infected sputum may spread to cause disease in new regions of the lungs. In patients who are receiving chemotherapy, the same thing is true as long as the sputum remains positive, though the degree of infectiousness is rapidly reduced. Even when the sputum is negative, an open cavity is a liability. We know that some of these cavities are truly healed, but in many cases the healing is incomplete, and living tubercle bacilli persist in the cavity wall. We know also that the relapse rate is higher in those patients who have open cavities than in those whose cavities have closed, even though the sputum is negative (7).

When cavities persist for more than six months after chemotherapy has been started, and the sputum remains positive, the cavity-bearing area should be resected if the patient's general condition justifies it. There is some risk involved in doing a resection in the presence of positive sputum, but this is minimal if the bacilli are still susceptible to the drugs which are being used or if a new and effective drug is added. As to patients who are "open-negative" (who have open cavities but negative sputum), the prolonged or indefinite use of isoniazid diminishes the risk of relapse to a low level, and resection has the disadvantage of reducing further the already reduced pulmonary function. In these "open-negative" patients resection should be reserved for patients with localized disease and excellent pulmonary function, and for patients who cannot be trusted to take isoniazid regularly for a long time.

Bed rest has only a limited place in the treatment of chronic pulmonary tuberculosis. The basis of treatment is chemotherapy, and chemotherapy is only effective against active, multiplying tubercle bacilli. Theoretically, bed rest reduces bacterial growth and multiplication, and to this extent actually reduces the effectiveness of the antituberculosis drugs. Clinical studies indicate that bed rest, used in conjunction with good chemotherapy, neither lessens nor enhances the effect of the drugs to any detectable extent (8). Therefore, when good chemotherapy is being given, the patient need not have any restrictions placed on his normal activity. There are still a few indications for bed rest, however. The patient who is acutely ill, with fever and other evidence of toxicity, may make a more rapid recovery if he is treated by bed rest in addition to drugs. Bed rest is useful in the control of pulmonary hemorrhage. Bed rest is also useful when no effective chemotherapy is possible, because of hypersensitivity, toxicity, or intolerance to the drugs or because the patient's bacilli are resistant to the available drugs.

Though interruption of drug treatment is harmful, planned changes in treatment may be helpful. Some have recommended that alternating regimens should be used from the beginning, hoping that by using two pairs of drugs alternately a better result would be obtained than by using the same two drugs throughout, and that drug resistance would be indefinitely postponed. The most successful of these regimens employs daily streptomycin and pyrazinamide one month and isoniazid and PAS the next month. The results of treatment with such alternating regimens are very good (9).

There are other reasons why drug treatment should sometimes be changed. If the planned treatment proves to be ineffective, as shown by lack of improvement, worsening, or relapse after initial improvement, the drug regimen should be changed. If resistance develops to a drug while it is being used for treatment, one can usually predict that further treatment with that drug will be ineffective (isoniazid is an exception to this general rule) and another drug should be substituted. Drug toxicity is another reason for discontinuing one drug and substituting another; examples are vestibular disturbance due to daily streptomycin, or severe anorexia, nausea and vomiting due to PAS. Hypersensitivity to a drug sometimes requires that the drug be stopped; the commonest offender in this regard is PAS, which occasionally causes a febrile response or a severe skin reaction which makes it necessary to stop the drug at once.

A number of regimens are used in the treatment of chronic pulmonary tuberculosis, and these will now be evaluated.

1. Isoniazid alone.
2. Streptomycin and PAS.
3. Isoniazid and streptomycin.
4. Isoniazid and PAS.
5. Isoniazid, PAS and streptomycin.
6. Alternating regimens.
7. Secondary drugs.

The first regimen to be discussed is isoniazid alone, given usually in doses of 100 mg three times daily. This is an effective regimen, resulting in resolution of lesions and sputum conversion in many cases of pulmonary tuberculosis, and even causing improvement in many cases of such formidable complications as miliary tuberculosis. However, it does not produce optimal results even in cases of non-cavitary tuberculosis. Effective therapy with two drugs has been shown to produce better results, with respect to sputum conversion, x-ray clearing, and clinical improvement, and therapy with two drugs is therefore preferred (1). The use of isoniazid alone is satisfactory for chemoprophylaxis and for the continuation treatment of patients who have already had a long course of treatment with two drugs. Though it has been used successfully in the therapy of non-cavitary pulmonary lesions, it is an inferior regimen for the treatment of any form of chronic pulmonary tuberculosis.

Streptomycin and PAS likewise constitute an inferior regimen, though for a number of years it was the best treatment available for tuberculosis. The results of therapy with this regimen are fairly good, but not as good as those obtained with two-drug regimens which employ isoniazid. Streptomycin is given in doses of 1 gm daily, and PAS in doses of 4 gm three times daily. Since daily streptomycin causes loss of vestibular function to some patients and hearing loss to some patients, about 10 per cent of patients cannot take this drug so frequently or in these doses. These can usually take this drug twice weekly, or daily in doses of 0.5 gm, without toxicity; and the reduced frequency or lower dosage does not greatly diminish the therapeutic efficacy of this regimen. Since isoniazid is our most valuable antituberculosis drug, and since it is desirable to make the first course of treatment as effective as possible, the combination of streptomycin and PAS is not the best choice for initial treatment. Yet it is fairly good treatment, and if isoniazid cannot be used for any reason, this somewhat inferior regimen may prove to be satisfactory.

Isoniazid and daily streptomycin is probably the most effective two-drug combination we have. The optimum dosage is—isoniazid, 100 mg three times daily, and streptomycin 1 gm daily. In the case of those patients who experience toxic manifestations to streptomycin in this dosage and frequency, the dose may be reduced to 0.5 gm daily or the frequency to 1 gm twice weekly, without much loss of efficacy. Though this combination is highly effective, streptomycin must be given intramuscularly, and outside of hospitals this creates some problems. Few clinics are prepared to give intramuscular injections oftener than twice weekly, and many patients find it inconvenient to go to their physicians or clinics for injections. As a result, regimens employing streptomycin are not widely used except in hospitals.

Isoniazid and PAS is the most widely used combination of drugs for initial treatment. It is highly efficacious in pulmonary and extrapulmonary tuberculosis, being only a trifle inferior to isoniazid and daily streptomycin. The usual dosage is—isoniazid 100 mg three times daily and PAS 4 gm three times daily. Higher doses of isoniazid are sometimes used, especially if there is partial resistance to this drug or if the drug is being rapidly inactivated. If doses of isoniazid larger than 300 mg daily are employed, pyridoxine should be given concurrently to prevent the development of peripheral neuritis. This combination of drugs is highly efficacious, inexpensive, low in toxicity and, being taken by mouth, it can be entirely self-administered. It is therefore logical to start treatment with this combination of drugs.

Case Report

This white man, thirty-nine years old, had had a slight morning cough and expectoration for about a year. In December 1963, the cough became more severe and the sputum more copious, and in the next month he experienced fever and night sweats and lost 10 pounds in weight. He was admitted to the hospital on January 10, 1964. Examination showed an underweight white man, both acutely and chronically ill. His temperature was 103° F. X-ray of the chest showed consolidation of the entire right upper lobe, with multiple cavities; planigrams confirmed the presence of several cavities ranging in size from 0.5 cm to 3 cm in diameter. The sputum was positive for acid-fast bacilli, both on concentration and culture. The tubercle bacilli were fully susceptible to streptomycin, isoniazid and PAS.

On January 11, 1964, chemotherapy was begun, and this consisted of isoniazid 100 mg three times daily and PAS 4 gm three times daily. His temperature gradually subsided, being normal for the first time on January 28, 1964. Thereafter the tempera-

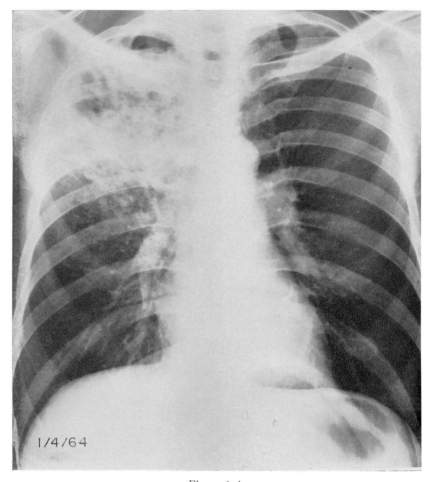

Figure 1-A

ture remained normal. Sputum volume gradually diminished, and the sputum culture was last positive on March 18. The sputum remained positive longer on concentration, but even by this technique the last positive report was dated July 1. Thereafter monthly concentrates and culture were all negative. Serial x rays showd rather spectacular clearing of the exudative component of the disease of the right upper lobe, but the cavities persisted. Planigrams on September 29, 1964 still showed multiple cavities, ranging in size from 1.5 cm to 3 cm in the markedly shrunken right upper lobe. Resectional surgery was therefore recommended, but the patient refused to accept this. On March

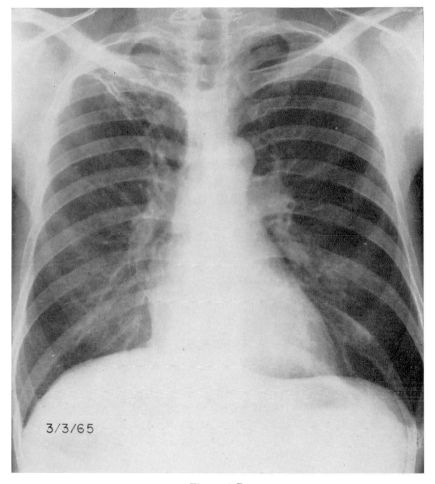

3/3/65

Figure 1-B

5, 1965, he was discharged with a work tolerance of eight hours daily. He is to continue isoniazid and PAS until he has taken this medication for a total of two years, and thereafter will continue isoniazid alone for a long time. He is working steadily as a cab driver, is taking his medication faithfully, and feels well.

The triple-drug combination—isoniazid 100 mg three times daily, PAS 4 gm three times daily, and streptomycin 1 gm daily—is highly effective. It is only a little more effective than the isoniazid and PAS combination, but is considerably more toxic. It is recommended in life-threatening tuberculosis. It is also justified at the beginning of treatment, when it is most important that treatment be rapidly successful. This regimen also ensures that if initial resistance exists to one drug the patient will nevertheless be receiving treatment with two effective drugs. When the laboratory tests have been reported, treatment may be continued with two drugs which have been shown to be effective. If possible these should be isoniazid and PAS.

Case Report

This patient was well until the age of fifty. In February, 1963, he noticed cough and expectoration, and soon afterward he became acutely ill, with fever, night sweats, weakness, weight

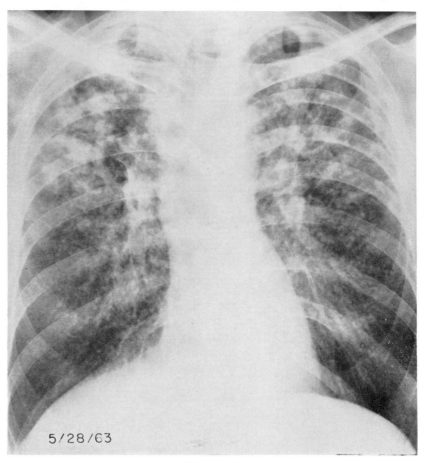

5/28/63

Figure 2-A

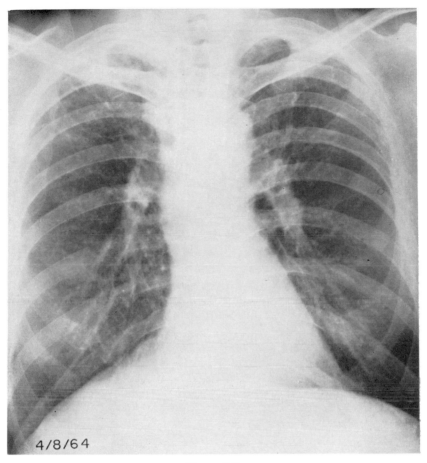

4/8/64

Figure 2-B

loss and dyspnoea. By May 1963, he had constant sore throat and pain on swallowing. The diagnosis of pulmonary tuberculosis and tuberculous laryngitis was made, and on May 27, 1963, he was admitted to the hospital.

Examination showed an undernourished, chronically ill white man, with a temperature of 102.4° F and with marked hoarseness. Examination of the larynx showed edema of the vocal cords and thickening of the left aryepiglottic fold, with a small ulcer. The diagnosis of tuberculous laryngitis was confirmed by biopsy. Chest roentgenograms showed extensive diffuse infiltration throughout both lungs, with cavitation in both upper lobes. Sputum was positive for acid-fast bacilli on concentrate and culture; the bacilli were completely susceptible to streptomycin, isoniazid and PAS.

Chemotherapy was started on May 28, 1963. This consisted of streptomycin 1 gm daily for forty-two days, and isoniazid 100 mg three times daily, and PAS 4 gm three times daily for two years. On this treatment he did very well. His temperature gradually came down to 99° F by June 13 and has been normal ever since. Appetite improved immediately, and he rapidly regained the weight he had lost; within one month he had gained 15 pounds and within six months he had gained thirty-three pounds. His sore throat and dysphagia disappeared within ten days and his hoarseness within two months. His sputum diminished strikingly in quantity. Sputum was last positive on concentration on June 12, 1963 and on culture on July 8, 1963; thereafter, monthly examinations were all negative. The x rays of the chest showed satisfactory clearing of the exudative lesions during the first six months, after which there was no further change. Planigrams on February 11, 1964 showed no residual cavitation. His physical activity was increased until he was doing the equivalent of a full day's work. He was discharged on June 3, 1964, and returned at once to full-time work as a foreman in a warehouse. He continued to take his isoniazid and PAS for a full two years, and has remained well.

This case demonstrates an excellent response to chemotherapy in spite of very extensive pulmonary tuberculosis complicated by tuberculous laryngitis.

Alternating regimens have been suggested as a means of providing maximum effectiveness with minimum risk of development of resistant tubercle bacilli. Two drugs are used for a period of time, then a second combination of two drugs is substituted. The two combinations are alternated monthly or every two months. Theoretically this arrangement has much to recommend it. Studies have shown alternating regimens to be highly effective. Streptomycin 1 gm daily and pyrazinamide 1 gm three times daily, alternating with isoniazid 100 mg three times daily and PAS 4 gm three times daily, is a highly effective combination.

Secondary drugs must sometimes be used, even in original treatment. They may be needed because primary resistance exists to the basic drugs, or because of hypersensitivity or toxicity. The principles of good treatment are the same as for primary drugs. Two effective drugs should be used, and they should be used for a long time. The secondary drugs are in general more toxic, less effective and more expensive than the basic drugs. Still, if the primary drugs cannot be used, an excellent result can often be obtained by the use of the secondary drugs.

Case Report

This white man, thirty-six years old, noticed weakness and fatigue during the early summer of 1963. By August 1963, his appetite was poor, he was losing weight, he had night sweats, and he had a slight but productive cough. He continued working until a pulmonary hemorrhage on October 4 forced him to go

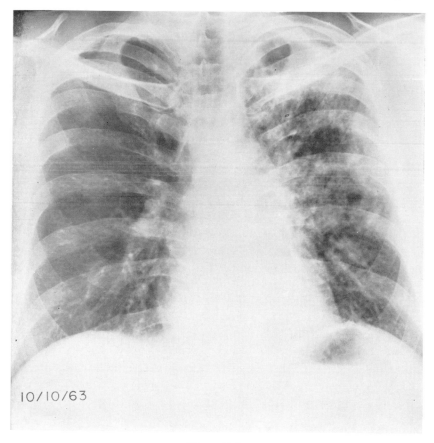

10/10/63

Figure 3-A

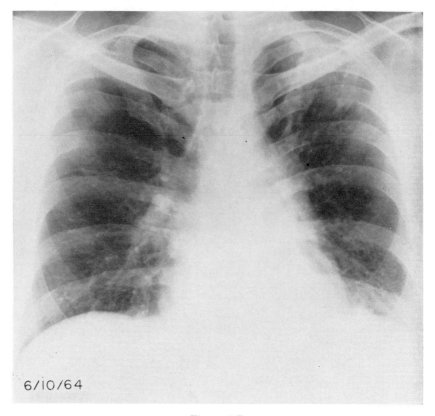

6/10/64

Figure 3-B

to his physician. The diagnosis of pulmonary tuberculosis was made, and on October 10 he was admitted to the hospital. Examination showed that he weighed 164 pounds (his average weight had been 180 pounds), and his temperature was 100.6° F. X ray of the chest revealed a dense, diffuse infiltrate in the upper half of the left lung, with a cavity 4.5 cm in diameter. The sputum was positive for acid-fast bacilli both on smear and culture, and susceptibility tests showed that the bacilli were fully susceptible to isoniazid, streptomycin, PAS, cycloserine and capreomycin.

Chemotherapy was started on October 22, 1963, the drugs employed being capreomycin 1 gm daily, and PAS 4 gm daily. The reason for the choice of these drugs was the desire to study the effectiveness of this combination in man; its effectiveness in experimental animals had already been established. On this regimen he did well. His appetite improved, he gained 25 pounds in weight, and his sputum become negative immediately; his first post-treatment sputum culture, on November 26, 1963, was negative, as were all subsequent smears and cultures. Serial chest x rays showed good steady clearing, and even the large cavity was no longer seen after February, 1964. He was discharged on September 25, 1964, able to return to his job full-time. Since his discharge he has been taking isoniazid and PAS under the supervision of the State Clinic, has worked steadily, and has remained well.

Summary

1. Two or more drugs should be used simultaneously.
2. Both drugs should be clinically effective. Bacteriological resistance should not exist against either of them.
3. Drug treatment should be uninterrupted.
4. Drug treatment should be prolonged.
5. Drugs should be changed if they are ineffective or toxic.
6. The basic drugs, isoniazid, streptomycin and PAS, are less toxic than the secondary drugs, and the first two are highly effective. The combinations isoniazid — PAS and isoniazid — streptomycin are excellent regimens.
7. Alternating regimens (such as streptomycin — pyrazinamide alternating with isoniazid   PAS, each pair of drugs being used for a month) have been shown to be highly effective.
8. Secondary drugs, such as cycloserine, viomycin, pyrazinamide, ethionamide, capreomycin and kanamycin, should be used if there is primary resistance to the basic drugs or if these drugs cannot be used because of toxicity or hypersensitivity. Any two-drug combination may be used, except that streptomycin, viomycin, capreomycin and kanamycin should not be used together because they have similar toxicities.

REFERENCES

1. SCHWARTZ, W. S.: Isoniazid alone compared with isoniazid and PAS in the treatment of minimal and non-cavitary, moderately advanced previously untreated pulmonary tuberculosis. *Trans. 20th Research Conference Pulmonary Diseases*, p. 75, 1961.

2. *Handbook of Tuberculosis Laboratory Methods,* Veterans Administration-Armed Forces Cooperative Study on the Chemotherapy of Tuberculosis, 1962. Superintendent of Documents, U. S. Government Printing Office, Washington 25, D. C.
3. Chemotherapy of tuberculosis in adults, A statement of the Committee on Therapy. *Amer. Rev. Resp. Dis., 92*:508, 1965.
4. Hobby, G. L., Lenert, T. F., Maier, J., O'Malley, P.: Primary drug resistance. *Amer. Rev. Resp. Dis., 91*:30, 1965.
5. Chaves, A. A.: Pulmonary tuberculosis. *Mod. Treat., 1*:330, 1964.
6. Fox, W.: The chemotherapy and epidemiology of tuberculosis. *Lancet, 2*:473, 1962.
7. Tuberculosis Chemotherapy Trials Committee, Tuberculosis Research Unit, Medical Research Council, Long-term chemotherapy in the treatment of chronic pulmonary tuberculosis with cavitation. *Tubercle, 43*:201, 1962.
8. Brace, A. A., and Spriggs, E. A.: Bed rest and institutional treatment in pulmonary tuberculosis. *Amer. Rev. Resp. Dis., 90*:183, 1964.
9. Corpe, R. F., and Blalock, F. A.: Alternating regimens of streptomycin-pyrazinamide, isoniazid-para-aminosalicylic acid at Battey State Hospital. *Amer. Rev. Resp. Dis., 90*:262, 1964.

Chapter VIII

RETREATMENT OF CHRONIC PULMONARY TUBERCULOSIS

RETREATMENT SHOULD very seldom be necessary if the first course of drug treatment has been adequate. It is when treatment has been interrupted, or discontinued too soon, that relapse is likely to occur and retreatment becomes necessary. Unfortunately, a high percentage of patients who are admitted to a hospital for the treatment of tuberculosis have already had unsuccessful drug treatment either at home or during a previous hospitalization. At the Butler Veterans Administration Hospital, 55 per cent of patients newly admitted for tuberculosis have had previous treatment. The principles of treatment are no different, whether retreatment or original treatment is involved. However, retreatment is more difficult, requires more laboratory control, and is less likely to be successful.

Retreatment should be begun, and carried on for a considerable period of time, in a hospital. Much laboratory work must be done to determine which drugs are effective, and if the secondary drugs are used, much laboratory work must be done so that early toxic manifestations can be recognized. It is of the utmost importance that the prescribed drugs be taken regularly, and the fact that the patient requires retreatment suggests that his drug intake during his first course of treatment was either irregular or of insufficient duration. Hospitalization permits the performance of drug-susceptibility testing, and the performance of tests which may demonstrate early drug toxicity, and offers an opportunity to educate the patient in the necessity of taking his drugs with complete regularity. All of these things can be done at home, but they can be done much better in a hospital.

As in original treatment, effective retreatment requires two drugs to which the tubercle bacilli are susceptible. It is desirable to have susceptibility tests done at the outset for all available drugs. While awaiting the results of these tests, isoniazid should be given along with two other drugs which have either not been used before or to which the patient's tubercle bacilli have recently been shown to be susceptible. When susceptibility tests have become available, the treatment may be changed. Isoniazid should be continued, and it should be accompanied by two drugs to which the tubercle bacilli are susceptible. If streptomycin and PAS are still effective, these are the drugs of choice. If resistance has developed to either or both of these drugs, a selection must be made from among the secondary drugs. Many are available—cycloserine, viomycin, pyrazinamide, ethionamide, capreomycin, ethambutol, kanamycin, thiocarbanidin and the thiosemicarbazones. There are no incombatibilities between these drugs. Streptomycin, viomycin, capreomycin and kanamycin have similar toxicities, so they should not be used together. Except for this, any combination of basic and secondary antituberculosis drugs can be used successfully (1) (2) (3) (4) (5) (6).

Isoniazid may be used successfully, even if the laboratory reports indicate that the bacilli are resistant to it. There is considerable evidence that, in the case of isoniazid, resistance in the test tube does not necessarily mean ineffectiveness clinically. Isoniazid may therefore be used to advantage, no matter how long it has been used before and no matter how complete the *in vitro* resistance has been shown to be (7). However, the drug should not be relied on as one of the two effective drugs that must be used, but should be used in addition to them.

As to the number of effective drugs that should be used, there should not be less than two. Some use a larger number (8) and as many as five or six drugs have been used at a time (9). The secondary drugs are in general much more toxic than the basic drugs, however, and the use of more than two such drugs at a time greatly increases the toxicity without a comparable increase in therapeutic efficacy. It is probably best to use the secondary drugs two at a time along with isoniazid.

It must be remembered that most of the secondary drugs are rather toxic, and also that strains of bacilli resistant to them tend to emerge in a few months, so that effective therapy with most secondary drug combinations is of short duration unless the sputum promptly becomes negative. For this reason, excisional surgery should be considered early. Persistent cavitation in the presence of persistently or intermittently positive sputum is a strong indication for resectional surgery. Residual cavitation in the presence of bacteriological relapse is likewise a strong indication for resection.

If resection is to be performed, it should be done early, while the drugs are still effective. Before surgery, it is best to administer the new drug combination for a month or two, in an effort to convert the sputum and minimize the postoperative complications. Even so, postoperative complications are common because the therapeutic efficacy of these regimens is relatively low. For this reason it is best to limit resectional surgery to lobectomy or occasional pneumonectomy; postoperative complications are especially common when segmental or subsegmental resections are done under cover of the secondary drugs.

In retreatment, even more than in original treatment, prolonged use of drugs is desirable. After the sputum has become negative, the drugs should be continued unchanged for at least one year and preferably longer. This creates a problem since, because of expense and possible toxicity, most of the secondary drugs are not available through clinics, and few private physicians are willing to take responsibility for their use. Most of the drug toxicity takes place in the early months of therapy, but the hepatic toxicity of pyrazinamide and the psychoses occasionally caused by cycloserine may occur at any time during the course of treatment. As a result, adequate retreatment often requires prolonged hospitalization. Some outpatient clinics are now prepared to supervise treatment with any drug combination that has been started in the hospital and to provide the necessary drugs, and when this is true, the patients may be discharged much earlier. Even after an adequate period of successful treatment with the secondary drugs (one to two years after the sputum becomes negative), isoniazid should be given for an additional two years or more. In spite of the most adequate treatment, relapses are common in this type of disease.

If a course of retreatment employing secondary drugs seems unsuccessful—that is, cavities remain open, sputum remains positive, and there is little clearing by x ray—the regimen should nevertheless be continued usually for six months or longer, because a favorable response to these drugs may take longer than a similar response to the basic drugs (10). If there is worsening of the tuberculous disease clinically or by x ray, if the laboratory reports that the tubercle bacilli are resistant to the new drugs, or if there is significant drug toxicity, the secondary drug combination must be stopped and a new combination employed. Usually this means the substitution of two previously unused drugs for the two secondary drugs currently employed. If substitutions are made one at a time, it is likely that partial resistance will exist to the drug which is retained. The new combination will therefore be only partially effective from the start, and resistance will rapidly develop to the new drug, rendering it also ineffective. It is best to make drug substitutions two at a time.

Retreatment is necessary in two situations: treatment failures and relapses (11). Treatment failure exists when a patient has received treatment for tuberculosis but still has active disease. A relapse is a reactivation of the disease after a period of inactivity (11).

Retreatment of patients who have suffered treatment failure requires an evaluation of previous drug intake, the presence or absence of cavitation, the extent and distribution of disease, the stability or progressive nature of the lesion, and the resistance or susceptibility of the tubercle bacilli to the basic and secondary drugs. Until laboratory studies of drug susceptibility are available, it may be assumed that the bacilli are susceptible to all drugs the patient has never received; this is not always true, as primary drug resistance sometimes exists, but this is not a frequent occurrence. If the previous course of treatment was too short, and the disease is not rapidly progressive, the patient may be treated with the same drugs he had received previously until drug-susceptibility tests have been completed.

If the disease is progressing rapidly, the substitution of two drugs never used before is safer than the use of the drugs previously taken. Once the drug-susceptibility of the bacilli is known, the physician should choose a combination of two drugs to which the bacilli are susceptible, to which isoniazid may be added. Any such combination should be effective. The physician should remember that 1) combinations including the basic drugs, isoniazid, streptomycin and PAS, are more effective and less toxic than those made up of the secondary drugs alone; 2) streptomycin, capreomycin, viomycin and kanamycin have similar toxicities, so no combination should contain more than one of these drugs; 3) the effectiveness of the secondary drugs is usually of short duration. If surgery is indicated, it should be carried out early in the course of retreatment.

The management of patients who have suffered a relapse is based on the same principles as in the case of treatment failure. The drugs selected for treatment must be drugs to which the patient's bacilli have been shown to be susceptible. However, since the bacilli of the patient who has relapsed are almost always resistant to the basic drugs, the chances of successful therapy are reduced.

If resistance to all the basic drugs is shown to exist, isoniazid may still be used, in addition to two secondary drugs of proven efficacy. Good combinations are cycloserine and viomycin, cycloserine and ethionamide, and pyrazinamide and ethionamide. It is vital that the drugs which are chosen should be drugs to which the patient's tubercle bacilli have been shown to be susceptible.

Retreatment cases vary greatly in the amount of previous treatment they have received, in the extent and duration of their disease, and in the susceptibility of their bacilli to the basic drugs. In general, they are much more difficult to treat successfully than original-treatment cases. In this difficult group of patients, long-term sputum conversion can be brought about in considerably more than 50 per cent of cases if the physician is resourceful and persistent, and if the patient is cooperative. Nevertheless, failure to convert the sputum and to return the patient to his community as a productive citizen is distressingly common in retreatment cases.

Patients who have suffered treatment failure or relapse are "hard-core" cases, and even the best retreatment program fails in a high percentage of cases. Also, a good retreatment program may not be acceptable to many of these patients. Some are alcoholic, and many are restless and undisciplined, so that refusal of drugs, surgery and prolonged hospitalization is common. As a result, there is a residuum of patients who continue to have active disease and who remain persistently infectious. Moreover, most of them excrete tubercle bacilli which are resistant to many antituberculosis drugs, so that people who become infected by them are severely handicapped. These persistently infectious patients must be prevented from spreading their tuberculosis to new victims.

Those who are intelligent and cooperative and who have satisfactory homes may be discharged to their homes when it is decided that nothing more can be done for them in the hospital. Many are so disabled as a result of pulmonary fibrosis and damaged pulmonary function that they require indefinite treatment in a hospital or nursing home. There remain a number of patients who must be isolated as long as they are infectious, not only in their own interest but also in the interest of the public health. They are not numerous but they constitute a serious problem. If they are allowed to leave the hospital, they are a source of infection. By persuasion, or if necessary by the compulsion of legal action through the local courts, they must be kept from infecting people in their communities. There are still about 50,000 new cases of active tuberculosis in the United States each year. Known cases of active tuberculosis who escape from supervision are an important source of infection.

Case Report

This patient was a prisoner-of-war in Germany in 1944. The diagnosis of pulmonary tuberculosis was made in 1947, and in the next few years he was treated by bedrest and left pneumothorax. In 1953, he received streptomycin and PAS for two months, but this was discontinued when he left the hospital against medical advice. In several subsequent examinations, his tuberculosis was believed to be moderately-advanced but inactive.

In June 1959, at the age of forty-two, he returned to the hospital complaining of weakness and weight loss. Chest x ray showed an increase in the extent of the disease in the right upper lobe, and planigrams showed a cavity in the right apex. Sputum was positive for acid-fast bacilli both on smear and culture, and the organisms were susceptible to streptomycin, isoniazid and PAS. Chemotherapy, consisting of isoniazid and PAS, was begun on July 16, 1959. There was some improvement symptomatically but x rays did not change significantly, so a right upper lobectomy was performed on October 7, 1959. There were no complications. Sputum culture was positive on October 26 and 28. PAS was discontinued on October 29, 1959, because of gastrointestinal

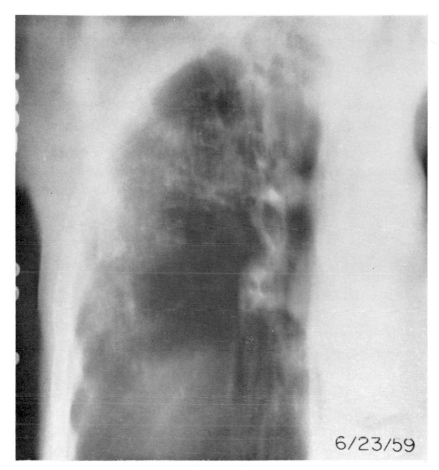

6/23/59

Figure 4-A

complaints, and streptomycin was substituted. Sputum was never again positive for acid-fast bacilli. He left the hospital against medical advice on February 11, 1960, but has continued to take isoniazid regularly. He has remained well, and is working steadily.

This case is an example of relapse after chemotherapy. The original chemotherapy was inadequate, having been given for only two months. Still, in the case of a patient with a record of both relapse and irregular discharges, it was felt desirable to treat not only with chemotherapy but with resection. The result was excellent.

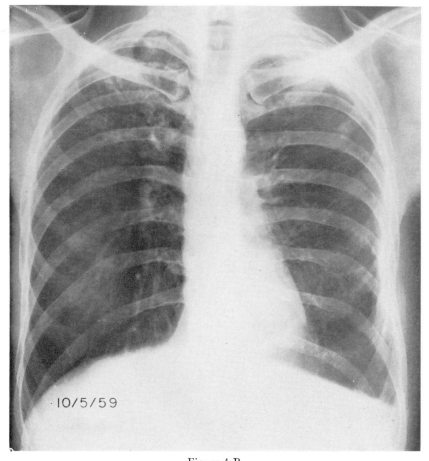

10/5/59

Figure 4-B

Case Report

In 1950, when he was forty-two years old, this white man was found to have pulmonary tuberculosis. He was an alcoholic and a restless individual, so that in the next eight years he had five hospital admissions, received streptomycin, PAS, isoniazid and pyrazinamide in various combinations, and had taken medication very irregularly when he was not hospitalized. He was admitted for the sixth time in January, 1958. Chest x rays at that time showed extensive bilateral fibrocavitary disease, with multiple cavities in both upper lobes. The sputum was positive for acid-fast bacilli, and the bacilli were resistant to streptomycin and

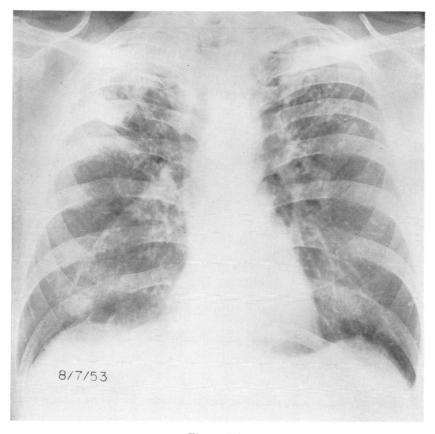

8/7/53

Figure 5-A

isoniazid and only partially susceptible to PAS. He was treated unsuccessfully with combinations of PAS, kanamycin and large doses of isoniazid (400 mgs three times daily). The sputum became negative while the patient was receiving kanamycin and PAS, but kanamycin was discontinued because of severe hearing loss, and sputum once more reverted to positive. On October 5, 1959, a regimen of cycloserine, pyridoxine and isoniazid was started. The dosage of cycloserine was 500 mg daily at first, but this was gradually increased so that by January 8, 1960, he was receiving 500 mg four times daily. On this regimen patient did well. Though there was no improvement by x ray, the sputum converted promptly. Sputum was last positive by smear on November 9, 1959, and by culture on September 14, 1959. All subsequent

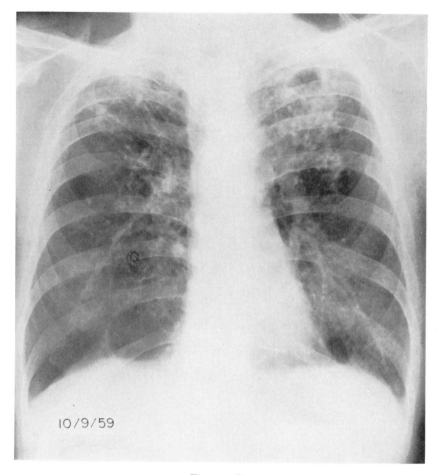

10/9/59

Figure 5-B

bacteriological examinations have been negative for acid-fast bacilli. Though he left the hospital against medical advice on March 10, 1960 and received no more cycloserine, and though his antituberculosis chemotherapy since then has been limited to isoniazid and PAS taken very irregularly, he has remained bacteriologically negative. He has been followed in a County Clinic, and has been in the hospital for nontuberculous diseases in 1963 and 1964. Innumerable sputum examinations by smear and culture have all been negative since November 1959.

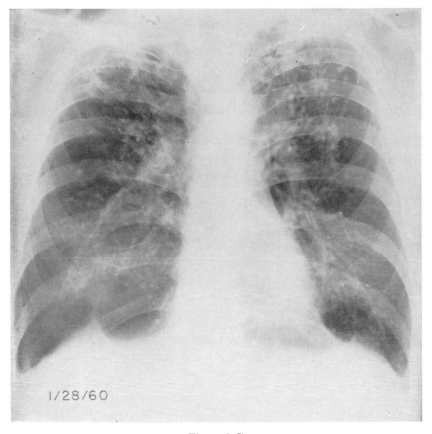

Figure 5-C

Case Report

In 1954, when this patient was thirty-one years old, he was found to have active pulmonary tuberculosis. During the next two years he was treated irregularly with dihydrostreptomycin and PAS and with streptomycin and PAS. He was admitted to the hospital in July, 1956. At that time, chest x ray showed extensive involvement of the right lung, with several large cavities. The sputum was positive for acid-fast bacilli, both on smear and culture, and the bacilli were resistant to isoniazid and partially resistant to streptomycin. An attempt was made to treat the patient according to the results of the drug-susceptibility tests, always

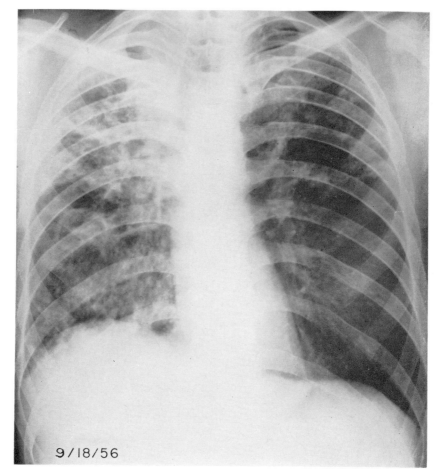

9/18/56

Figure 6-A

using two drugs to which the bacilli were susceptible. He was treated with varying combinations of isoniazid, PAS, streptomycin, pyrazinamide and kanamycin. Each combination was effective for a time, but then resistant strains of bacilli emerged and the disease progressed again. In April, 1959, treatment was changed to cycloserine and viomycin—cycloserine in doses beginning with 250 mg two times daily, rapidly increasing to 2000 mg daily in divided doses, and viomycin in doses of 2 gm twice weekly. On this regimen sputum volume decreased, the sputum smears and cultures were negative more often than they were

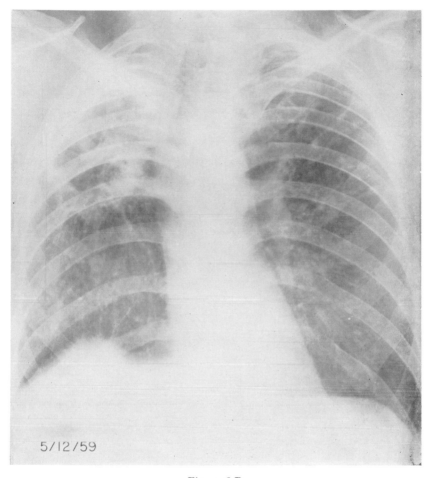

5/12/59

Figure 6-B

positive, and progression of disease stopped. After several months of stability, a pneumonectomy was performed on September 17, 1959. The cavities showed a high degree of healing, with considerable reepithelization. On September 27, 1959, patient had a transient psychosis during which he was suspicious and had delusions of persecution. It was feared that this might be a toxic reaction to cycloserine, so this drug was discontinued; and although the psychosis ended in a few days, the drug was never restarted. Chemotherapy for the next few months consisted of isoniazid and viomycin, and then he received isoniazid alone.

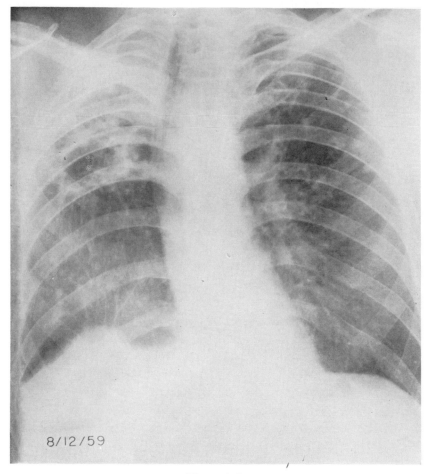

8/12/59

Figure 6-C

He has been observed periodically until May 10, 1965. He never again had a positive sputum and no disease has developed in the left lung.

This patient did not recover on the primary drugs, partly because of irregular treatment, and he did poorly on a succession of secondary drugs. His disease was finally stabilized by the use of a combination of drugs which he had never received before, cycloserine and viomycin. During this period of stability a pneumonectomy was successfully performed. He has had no evidence of active tuberculosis since.

SUMMARY

1. Retreatment is seldom necessary if the first course of treatment is adequate. It is needed in cases when the original treatment has failed, and in relapses.

2. About half of the patients now admitted to a hospital for the treatment of tuberculosis have had previous treatment.

3. Retreatment is more difficult and less successful than original treatment. It should be begun in a hospital, and continued for a considerable period of time in a hospital.

4. At the beginning of a course of retreatment, the whole medical situation should be evaluated, the history of previous drug administration reviewed, the susceptibility of the tubercle bacilli to the various drugs determined, and a decision made as to the probable need for resectional surgery. Then an intelligent plan of treatment can be made, integrating surgery (if needed) into the overall therapy. If needed, surgery should be done early.

5. Retreatment, like original treatment, requires a combination of at least two drugs to which the bacilli are susceptible.

6. In retreatment, even more than in original treatment, it is important that the drugs be given for a long time. The successful combination of drugs should be given for a year or two after the sputum has become negative, and then isoniazid should be given for another two years or longer.

7. The drugs used in retreatment are usually more toxic and less effective than the basic drugs.

8. The percentage of failures is high in retreatment.

REFERENCES

1. PETTY, T. L., AND MITCHELL, R. S.: Successful treatment of advanced isoniazid-and streptomycin-resistant pulmonary tuberculosis with ethionamide, pyrazinamide, and isoniazid. *Amer. Rev. Resp. Dis., 86*:503, 1962.

2. AQUINAS, M.: Pyrazinamide and ethionamide in the treatment of pulmonary tuberculosis in Hong Kong. *Tubercle, 44*:76, 1963.

3. CHAVES, A. D., ABELES, H., AND ROBINS, A. B.: Ethionamide-cycloserine therapy for ambulatory patients with pulmonary tu-

berculosis unresponsive to standard drugs. *Amer. Rev. Resp., Dis., 88*:254, 1963.

4. RUIZ, R. C.: D-Cycloserine in the treatment of pulmonary tuberculosis resistant to the standard drugs. *Dis. Chest, 45*:181, 1964.

5. SCHLESS, J. M., ALLISON, R. F., INGLIS, R. M., WHITE, E. F., AND TOPPERMAN, S.: The use of ethionamide in combined drug regimens in the retreatment of isoniazid-resistant pulmonary tuberculosis. *Amer. Rev. Resp. Dis., 91*:728, 1965.

6. OKA, S., KONNO, K., KUDO, S., MUNAKATA, K., YAMAGUCHI, E., AND OIZUMI, K.: Clinical studies on ethambutol. *Amer. Rev. Resp. Dis., 91*:762, 1965.

7. WOLINSKY, E., AND KAPUR, V. N.: Effect of withdrawal of isoniazid in chronic, stable, treatment-failure cases with drug-resistant tubercle bacilli. *Amer. Rev. Resp. Dis., 81*:941, 1960.

8. PINES, A.: The fate of patients with drug-resistant tubercle bacilli and pulmonary tuberculosis. *Brit. J. Dis. Chest. 56*:163, 1962.

9. BERNARD, E., ISRAEL, L., PARIENTE, D., AND WEIL, B.: Resultats favorables de la chimiotherapie antibacillaire sextuple dans les tuberculoses pulmonaires inveterees. *Rev. Tuberc. (Paris), 27*:197, 1963.

10. CHAVES, A. D.: Pulmonary tuberculosis. *Mod. Treat., 1*:330, 1964.

11. Committee on therapy of the American Thoracic Society, The chemotherapeutic management of treatment failures and relapses in pulmonary tuberculosis. *Amer. Rev. Resp. Dis., 82*:751, 1960.

Chapter IX

EXTRAPULMONARY TUBERCULOSIS

THE PRIMARY tuberculosis infection is usually pulmonary, but in a small percentage of cases (less than 5 per cent) it may be extrapulmonary. Occasionally, primary sites of infection outside the lungs are the alimentary tract, skin, conjunctiva and genitals.

Case Report

This patient was a laryngologist, twenty-nine years of age, with a negative skin reaction to tuberculin. In 1946, he began to take care of patients with active pulmonary tuberculosis. He was meticulous about wearing a mask whenever he examined or treated tuberculous patients. About six months after this exposure began, he noticed a small nodule with a small, painless, unhealing ulcer on the left cheek, where the lower string of the mask rubbed against the skin over the mandible. The nodule reached a maximum size of 8 mm and was never painful or tender, and the ulcer was never more than 3 mm in diameter. At first he ignored this lesion, but within a few weeks there was a soft, fluctuant, nontender swelling at the angle of the left jaw. Five cc of pus was aspirated from this swelling, and acid-fast bacilli were demonstrated by both smear and culture. He had no fever or other evidence of constitutional illness. He remained on duty, and was given a course of chemotherapy consisting of streptomycin, 1 gm intramuscularly daily and PAS 4 gm by mouth three times daily for ninety days. Today therapy would be continued much longer. The ulcer healed within two weeks, but the swelling regressed much more slowly. Eight weeks after the appearance of the nodule, the tuberculin test was repeated and was found positive. Ten years later the patient was reexamined; he had remained well, and had no evidence of tuberculosis at the site of the original lesion or anywhere else in the body. The lesion of the skin and of the draining glands at the angle of the jaw constituted a typical primary tuberculous complex, though in an unusual location.

[117]

Case Report

This patient was a seaman aged twenty-three. In July 1958, he developed a lesion on the foreskin and swelling of the left inguinal lymph glands. Biopsy of the foreskin showed an ulcerative granulomatous lesion, and incision of the glands revealed caseous material. Smears and cultures of this caseous material demonstrated acid-fast bacilli. Isoniazid and PAS were started at once. Studies showed no evidence of tuberculosis elsewhere in the genitourinary tract, in the lungs or elsewhere in the body. The lesion on the penis healed within a few weeks. Drugs were continued for two years. The patient was last seen in July 1964, at which time he showed no evidence of tuberculosis anywhere in his body. This case illustrated the occasional extrapulmonary location of the primary tuberculous complex.

Primary tuberculosis can only occur, of course, in locations which can be infected from outside the body. The mode of infection may be by inhalation, ingestion, contamination of the skin, or penetration through the skin. Primary extrapulmonary tuberculosis usually occurs as a result of the latter three routes (ingestion, contamination of the skin, or penetration through the skin), and is becoming rather uncommon. It should be suspected when the tuberculin reaction is positive, the chest x ray is negative, and there is a chronic ulcer accompanied by a painless, nontender swelling of the regional lymph glands. The diagnosis can only be made with certainty by finding tubercle bacilli in the ulcer at the portal of entry or in pus or caseous material from the regional lymph node. In the case of primary intestinal tuberculosis, a rarity now that bovine tuberculosis has almost disappeared and much rarer in adults than in children, the diagnosis cannot be made with certainty without surgery. It can be strongly suspected if the tuberculin reaction is positive and the patient has marked swelling of the abdominal glands and a negative chest x ray. Primary extrapulmonary tuberculosis should be treated with two drugs. The most common combination of effective drugs is isoniazid 100 mg three times daily and PAS 4 gm three times daily; chemotherapy should be continued for a year or longer.

Though the primary tuberculous infection usually occurs in the lungs, we have seen that at some stage early in its development tuberculosis is often a generalized disease. The wide-spread dissemination of tubercle bacilli throughout the body in the weeks following primary infection has been described in the chapter on Pathogenesis. The extrapulmonary foci of infection which result from this dissemination are usually contained by the body's defenses and eventually healed, but in a small percentage of untreated cases significant disease develops. By the time the extrapulmonary disease becomes manifest, the primary infection, whether in the lungs or elsewhere, may not be apparent, so the extrapulmonary tuberculosis appears to be localized rather than part of a widely disseminated disease. Various types of extrapulmonary tuberculosis will be discussed.

MILIARY TUBERCULOSIS

Acute miliary tuberculosis results when a large number of tubercle bacilli are discharged into the circulation simultaneously. This may happen when a caseous focus adjacent to a blood vessel involves the vessel wall, invades the intima, and then discharges large numbers of tubercle bacilli in one or a series of showers. The source may also be an intimal tubercle, which developed following an earlier bloodstream dissemination. Whatever the source, the tubercle bacilli which are discharged into the blood-stream lodge in capillaries and form tubercles. These may heal spontaneously, or they progress to caseation.

Acute miliary tuberculosis usually occurs in the first few months after the primary infection, though it may occur later. The patient is acutely ill, with fever and usually an elevated white blood count. Usually the tuberculin test is positive in the earliest phase of the disease, but later the reaction becomes negative. Without the use of the antituberculosis drugs the disease almost always progresses, the local lesions caseate, and the fever remains high or remittent. Most untreated patients die within a few months, usually after developing tuberculous meningitis.

Chemotherapy, and especially therapy which includes isoniazid, has dramatically changed the course of acute miliary tuberculosis. On effective chemotherapy, the progression of tubercles is stopped, and the patients usually make a good recovery. Caseous foci which have already developed usually heal, but sometimes tubercle bacilli may persist for a long time in these foci, and occasionally they may cause disease at a later time. The mortality, which was once nearly 100 per cent, is now very low except in that group of neglected patients whose treatment is not started until they are at the point of death (1).

Therapy should be started as soon as the diagnosis is made or is strongly suspected. It is desirable to begin treatment with three drugs. An effective combination consists of streptomycin 1 gm daily intramuscularly, isoniazid 100 mg or more three times daily by mouth, and PAS 4 gm three times daily by mouth. Treatment should be continued for two years or longer, though the frequency of streptomycin administration may be reduced to twice weekly after the first few months, especially if there is evidence of hearing loss or vestibular damage. The steroid hormones are seldom needed, but may be helpful if used for a few weeks when chemotherapy is begun.

This discussion has been concerned with acute miliary tuberculosis resulting from a single massive seeding of tubercle bacilli into the bloodstream from a caseous focus. Sometimes the seedings are less massive and are repeated many times. If the patient is not overwhelmed by the disease during its early months, distant foci may result from these seedings in many parts of the body. Without therapy with the antituberculosis drugs the course was almost always downhill, the patient eventually dying with caseous tuberculous lesions of varying sizes throughout the body. Chemotherapy, employing the same drugs and dosages listed in the last paragraph, will usually stop further dissemination and permit healing of the existing caseous foci.

Since chemoprophylaxis and chemotherapy have been widely used, miliary tuberculosis has become much rarer than it was formerly. Predisposing factors are advanced age and chronic alcoholism (2).

TUBERCULOUS MENINGITIS AND TUBERCULOMA

Tuberculous meningitis seldom develops as a result of the direct seeding of tubercle bacilli on the meninges by way of the bloodstream. Rather it results from growth of a caseous focus in the brain or skull which finally involves the meninges and deposits in the cerebrospinal fluid not a few tubercle bacilli but a great many in a sudden catastrophe (3). The caseous focus is, of course, the result of an earlier hematogenous seeding. This concept of the origin of tuberculous meningitis is important, because it enables us to understand the sudden origin of the disease and its rapid evolution, and because it gives us information which permits us to plan both intelligent prevention and treatment. Since the caseous focus which is the cause of the meningitis usually owes its origin to a hematogenous spread early in the course of the primary infection, almost always both the focus and the meningitis can be prevented by prophylactic isoniazid therapy given as soon as primary tuberculosis is recognized. Since the evolution of meningitis is rapid, and since the brain is involved early in the course of the disease, treatment must be started early and carried out intensively, not only to save life but to prevent irreparable damage to the brain and cranial nerves.

Tuberculous meningitis may begin either abruptly or insidiously. Fever, headache and vomiting are common complaints, and apathy is often noticed by the family. In young children, convulsions sometimes occur early in the course of the disease. In a week, or perhaps longer, all the patient's signs and symptoms have progressed, and in addition, neurological signs appear, indicating central nervous system involvement. At this time the patient is drowsy or irritable. At this time, too, neurological examination is likely to show a stiff neck, absent abdominal reflexes, and increased deep reflexes. Sometimes there is mental confusion at this stage. About the beginning of the third week, there is restlessness and confusion which soon progress to unresponsiveness and coma. There is almost never spontaneous recovery from tuberculous meningitis. If effective therapy is not given, the mortality is almost 100 per cent. The diagnosis of tuberculosis is questionable in those few cases of meningitis reported to have recovered without chemotherapy.

Tuberculous meningitis is never limited to the meninges, but always, to a greater or lesser extent, involves the brain. We have seen that it usually begins as a result of the extension of a caseous focus in the brain. As it develops, it involves most extensively the area around the brain stem. The exudate around the base of the brain often obstructs the flow of cerebrospinal fluid from the cisterns, causing internal hydrocephalus. This exudate also causes frequent involvement of the cranial nerves, with impairment of vision, hearing, or the extra-ocular muscles. In the brain, itself, there may be exudation, the formation of caseous tubercles, and extensive tuberculous involvement of arterial walls. The latter may cause total obstruction of arteries, with softening of those portions of the brain supplied by those arteries. It can be seen that the clinical picture of tuberculous meningitis may be extremely variable, depending on the extent and location of the brain lesions, and on the extent and location of the exudation around the brain stem. It can also be seen that it is of the greatest importance to start chemotherapy early, because some of the lesions (e.g., areas of infarction due to obstruction of cerebral arteries), may be prevented but are irreversible once they have developed.

The diagnosis of tuberculous meningitis should be suspected when unexplained fever, headache, vomiting and apathy exist. The tuberculin test is usually positive, though anergy and a negative tuberculin reaction are common in the terminal stages of the disease. The chest x ray shows evidence of primary tuberculous infection in the great majority of cases. The spinal fluid is typically clear, with a few cells, an increased protein content, and reduced chlorides and glucose. The cells number from 5 to 300 per cu mm, and rarely the cell count rises to 1000. Most of the cells are lymphocytes, though very early in the course of the disease about half of the cells may be polymorphonuclear leucocytes. The spinal fluid protein is almost always elevated, and as the disease progresses the protein tends to increase; it is common to find levels of 300 mg per 100 ml and 1 gm or even 2 gm per 100 ml are not rare. The chlorides are often normal early in the disease, but are usually reduced later.

The glucose is usually reduced from the start, and the more advanced the disease, the lower the spinal fluid glucose becomes. When the fluid is allowed to stand, a pellicle forms, and bacteriological examination of this pellicle will often reveal a few tubercle bacilli. Culture of the spinal fluid will also show tubercle bacilli in many cases. Bacteriological proof is required to make a positive diagnosis of tuberculous meningitis, but treatment must be started in most cases before bacteriological proof is available. If the history and physical examination are suggestive of tuberculous meningitis, and if the laboratory examination of the cerebrospinal fluid gives results which are compatible with this disease, drug treatment should be started at once. A delay of a week or two, if the diagnosis of tuberculosis proves correct, may result in death or irreparable brain damage. It must be repeated: If the diagnosis of tuberculous meningitis is probable, treatment should be started at once, without waiting for proof.

The prognosis of the patient with tuberculous meningitis depends on the stage at which the diagnosis is made and effective treatment started. If treatment is started within a few days of the initial symptoms, the patient will almost always survive, and will suffer minimal brain damage or none at all. If treatment is started after there is evidence of brain damage or cranial nerve involvement, the patient's response is slower, there is more permanent brain damage, and some patients fail to recover. If treatment is delayed until coma develops, there is considerable danger of death, and those who recover run a considerable risk of having serious and permanent neurological defects. If chemotherapy is not given at all, there is almost no hope of recovery. Recent studies stress the frequency of residual neurological defects when treatment is started late (4) (5) and the generally good results of effective treatment (6) (7). Relapses are few after effective treatment (8).

Effective treatment consists of at least two, and usually three drugs, started as early in the course of the disease as possible and continued for two years or longer. A good program consists of streptomycin 1 gm intramuscularly daily, isoniazid 100 mg three times daily by mouth, and PAS 4 gm three times daily by mouth. Since streptomycin can pass through the inflamed meninges, and since isoniazid can enter the cerebrospinal fluid even when the meninges are normal, it is not necessary to give streptomycin intrathecally. Indeed, intrathecal streptomycin is not only unnecessary but is capable of causing neurological sequelae itself, so it is not recommended.

As to the use of steroids along with the antituberculosis drugs, there is some difference of opinion. Steroids reduce inflammation and exudation, and these actions may be helpful or harmful. In tuberculous meningitis, the effect of steroids is likely to do more good than harm. In cases in which the diagnosis is made early and treatment with the antituberculosis drugs is started early, there is usually no need for the steroid hormones. When the prognosis is less good, as when treatment is started late or when the patient is an infant, steroids may be life-saving or may prevent brain damage. It is good practice to give steroid therapy if the patient is in coma, if he already has neurologic signs when he is first seen, if he is less than one year old, if obstruction exists to the flow of spinal fluid, or if the meningitis does not respond well to the antituberculosis drugs alone.

In these situations the steroids should be given in doses sufficient to reduce the temperature to normal and to minimize symptoms. In adults the dose is usually 10 to 20 mg prednisone three times daily (or its equivalent), while children may be given 1 to 3 mg per kg body weight daily. Steroids should be continued at these levels for about a month, and then gradually tapered off. Steroids may be expected to produce quick symptomatic improvement and to speed up the rise in sugar content and the lowering of the protein content of the cerebrospinal fluid, but the main reasons they are given are to reduce toxicity, reduce the inflammatory exudate, prevent or relieve obstruction to the free flow of cerebrospinal fluid, and prevent damage to the brain. It is important never to give steroids unless effective antituberculosis drugs are given at the same time.

Case Report

This patient was a white man, thirty-five years of age, who was perfectly well until January, 1947. At that time he noticed cough, expectoration, weakness, loss of appetite and loss of weight, but was able to continue working. On July 10 he stopped working. He did not seem acutely ill, but his wife said he was apathetic, taking no interest in his home or surroundings. On July 12 he began to vomit, and this persisted. On July 17 he became confused. He was admitted to the hospital on July 18. Examination showed a man who was undernourished and who was both acutely and chronically ill, restless and thrashing about in bed. He was confused and disoriented. Temeprature was 99.8° F, the neck was stiff, the left pupil was dilated, there was a positive Kernig, and the abdominal reflexes were absent. The chest roentgenogram showed bilateral apical involvement with a small cavity on the right, but sputum examination failed to reveal acid-fast bacilli.

The cerebrospinal fluid was clear, with a cell count of 179 (100 per cent lymphocytes); the total protein was 77 mg per 100 ml, and the sugar was 25 mg per 100 ml. On standing, a pellicle formed on the fluid. Smear from the pellicle was negative for acid-fast bacilli, but the culture was reported positive after eight weeks' incubation.

Chemotherapy was started on July 18, and was continued for 120 days. He received streptomycin 2 gm daily intramuscularly and 0.05 gm daily intrathecally during this time. The temperature promptly came down to normal, the mental confusion gradually disappeared, and the pulmonary lesion rapidly improved. At first the cerebrospinal fluid cell count and protein rose, but soon they began to decline. Neuropsychiatric examinations on December 8, 1947, showed a positive Babinski on the right, moderate dysarthria, a markedly atactic gait, pronounced euphoria and impairment of judgment. On May 11, 1948, the spinal fluid cell count was 25 and the protein was 52 mg per 100 ml. He was discharged in September, 1948.

He was readmitted on February 14, 1949, with fever and severe headache. The cerebrospinal fluid now showed 423 cells (94 per cent lymphocytes) and a protein content of 350 mg per ml. Once more he received streptomycin 2 gm daily intramuscularly and 0.05 gm daily intrathecally for four months. He improved symptomatically, and on June 1, 1949, the spinal fluid cell count was 11 (81 per cent lymphocytes) and the protein content was 150 mg per 100 ml. He was discharged on February 4, 1950.

He has had no further relapses. Yearly contacts showed that he was able to work steadily, eight hours a day, until 1960. His only complaints were slight dizziness and a moderate hearing loss. His euphoria and poor judgment persisted. Though his physical health remained good, he became increasingly unreliable, the quality of his work deteriorated, and be was discharged by his employer for inefficiency in 1960.

This patient was treated inadequately, by present day standards. He received only one drug, the dose was large enough to produce significant toxicity and was given for too short a time to be fully effective, and the drug was given intrathecally, a route of administration which is now known to be both unnecessary and toxic. Nevertheless, even this inadequate treatment saved the patient's life. Since treatment was not started until there was already evidence of brain damage (as indicated by confusion and reflex changes), evidence of residual brain damage should not be surprising. If brain damage is to be prevented, treatment *must* be started early.

Tuberculomas of the brain result from the implantation and growth of tubercle bacilli in the brain in the period immediately following the primary infection. In most cases these caseous foci heal, causing minimal brain damage, and never again produce signs or symptoms of disease. In some cases they may progress, and in others they may remain dormant for a long time and then begin growing again. Some of these reach the meninges, causing tuberculous meningitis, while others cause signs and symptoms only by their presence. These latter tuberculomas are expanding, space-occupying brain lesions which are usually at first believed to be neoplastic. They may cause headache, increased intracranial pressure, epileptiform seizures and focal symptoms which vary according to the location of the lesion. Treatment is mainly the prolonged use of two antituberculosis drugs, followed by surgical removal if the signs and symptoms do not disappear. In those cases in which the mass is removed because of the diagnosis of brain tumor, the correct diagnosis being made later, prolonged chemotherapy should be given as soon as the diagnosis of tuberculosis is made. Tuberculomas of the brain have never been common, and are becoming increasingly rare.

Case Report

This man had an epileptic seizure at the age of forty-five. This was his first seizure. Examination showed far-advanced, active pulmonary tuberculosis with bilateral cavitation, and sputum was positive for acid-fast bacilli. He was treated with isoniazid and PAS, following which there was radiological improvement and sputum conversion. The seizures continued, however, and were associated with transient weakness of the left arm and leg. Neurological examination, electroencephalograms and angiograms showed a lesion in the right parietal lobe. This was removed surgically and found to be a caseous tuberculous focus about 1 cm in diameter.

GENITOURINARY TUBERCULOSIS

Genitourinary tuberculosis was formerly one of the more common forms of extrapulmonary tuberculosis, and although it is decreasing

in frequency, it is still seen from time to time. It is usually hematogenous in origin (though occasionally it develops by extension from
nearby structures), but by the time it becomes manifest the original
focus may have healed completely so that the disease in the genitourinary tract is the only detectable disease. It rarely heals without
chemotherapy.

Within the urinary tract, the primary location of tuberculosis is
almost always in the kidneys. The infection often travels downward,
involving the bladder, prostate, vesicles and epididymis but almost
never travels upward to the kidneys against the urinary flow. The
initial infection of the kidney usually heals entirely, but sometimes it
may progress to cause caseation and involvement of the kidney pelvis.
Sometimes, too, the initial renal infection becomes quiescent but does
not heal entirely; when this happens the small, dormant lesion may
become reactivated and cause progressive and destructive renal tuberculosis years later.

Hematuria is the commonest finding in renal tuberculosis, and
may be the only finding. When tuberculosis has progressed to involve
the ureter and bladder, there will also be frequency, dysuria and
pyuria. Cystoscopy will show inflammation of the bladder mucosa,
sometimes with ulceration. When tuberculosis of the bladder has
lasted for some time, the bladder wall is thickened and its capacity
is reduced. A urogram will show the extent and location of the
disease in the kidneys and ureters; it may demonstrate blunting of
the calyces (due to destruction of small amounts of adjoining renal
parenchyma), renal cavities (due to the formation and evacuation of
abscesses), and ureteral stricture. A definite diagnosis requires the
finding of acid-fast bacilli in the urine. For this purpose urine smears
or concentrates are worthless, as the acid-fast smegma bacillus is a
common contaminant. Reliance must be placed on the identification
of tubercle bacilli on culture or animal inoculation of a urine specimen. The identification of tubercle bacilli in the urine is proof of
tuberculosis of the genitourinary tract, as tubercle bacilli cannot pass
through the undamaged kidney (9).

The treatment of renal tuberculosis is fundamentally drug treatment. Rest in bed is more important in the treatment of renal tuberculosis than it is in pulmonary tuberculosis, so it is best to initiate
treatment in a hospital. So effective is drug treatment that nephrec-

tomy or hemi-nephrectomy is very rarely necessary. Even if stenosis of a ureter develops, resectional surgery is seldom necessary; these stenoses can be dilated, and they tend not to recur. Good chemotherapy requires three drugs given concurrently for two years or longer. The most desirable of these, as effective as any and less toxic than most, consists of:

Isoniazid	100 mg three times daily.
Streptomycin	1 gm daily, six to twelve weeks, then twice weekly.
PAS	4 gm three times daily.

If any of these drugs cannot be given because of toxicity or hypersensitivity, or if clinically or bacteriologically there is evidence that one of these drugs is ineffective, there are a number of other drugs which can serve as satisfactory substitutes. Among them are the following.

Cycloserine	250 mg twice daily.
Viomycin	2 gm twice weekly.
Pyrazinamide	1 gm three times daily.
Ethionamide	250 mg twice daily.
Capreomycin	1 gm daily.
Kanamycin	1 gm twice weekly.

Of these drugs, cycloserine is perhaps the most effective since it is concentrated in the renal tubules, and in these doses it is of low toxicity. Since streptomycin, viomycin, capreomycin and kanamycin have similar toxicities, and since their toxicities are additive, only one of them should be used in any combination of drugs. On a three-drug regimen about 97 per cent of patients have conversion of the urine, and there are few relapses after drug therapy is stopped (10). If urine cultures are persistently positive this usually means that resistant organisms are present; susceptibility tests should be done, and a drug combination of proven effectiveness should be substituted (11).

Genital tuberculosis may involve the prostate, seminal vesicles, testes and epididymides in males, and the Fallopian tubes and the uterus in females. Tuberculosis of the external genitalia is uncommon.

Genital tuberculosis may occur either as a result of blood-borne dissemination from a distant focus (usually in the lungs) or as a descending infection from a renal focus; in adult males it is most commonly secondary to renal disease.

Tuberculosis of the prostate produces few signs or symptoms, and is often undiscovered. It may be suspected when the prostate is nodular and the presence of tuberculosis elsewhere can be demonstrated. Similarly, tuberculosis of the seminal vesicles is not uncommon but is often undiagnosed because it produces no signs or symptoms. It usually occurs in conjunction with tuberculosis of the prostate, and rectal examination will disclose nodulation of the vesicles. Tuberculous epididymitis usually causes a nodular, painless, nontender swelling which gradually enlarges and involves the testis. If drug treatment is not given the swelling continues to progress, caseation occurs, and eventually multiple fistulas form. Less commonly, tuberculous epididymitis begins acutely rather than insidiously, and there is rapid swelling accompanied by pain and tenderness.

Tuberculous salpingitis is by far the most common form of genital tuberculosis in the female. It is often symptomless, and may be productive of menstural irregularity or sterility. Physical examination may show enlargement and slight tenderness of one or both tubes, and sterility may result if the tubes are occluded. The infection may spread from the tubes in either or both directions. If it spreads through the fimbriated end it may cause tuberculosis of the ovary or the pelvic peritoneum, and if it spreads medially it may result in a tuberculous endometritis.

The treatment of genital tuberculosis is similar to the treatment of tuberculosis of the urinary tract; three drugs should be given, starting as soon as the diagnosis is made and continuing for two years. Certain refractory foci, such as the prostate, may require much longer treatment (11). Surgery is limited to the resection of large residual masses of necrotic tissue. Genital tuberculosis can be prevented by the chemotherapy of primary tuberculosis. It can be cured by adequate chemotherapy of the genital disease. A good functional result depends on starting drug treatment early, before irreversible damage has been done.

Case Report

In 1947, when he was thirty-nine years old, this patient was found to have active pulmonary tuberculosis, with cavitation on the right and positive sputum. He received streptomycin, 2 gm daily for forty-two days with some benefit, but his sputum remained positive. A year later he noticed frequency and dysuria. The urine at that time was found to show red and white blood cells on microscopic examination, and the urine culture was positive for acid-fast bacilli. Cystoscopy showed ulceration of the bladder mucosa. The ureters were catheterized, and the urine from both kidneys proved to be positive for acid-fast bacilli. Retrograde pyelograms showed blunting of the calyces of both kidneys, more marked on the left than on the right. Examination showed that the prostate was involved too. Streptomycin 2 gm daily and PAS 4 gm three times daily were given, but after ten weeks the patient developed a skin rash and streptomycin had to be stopped. PAS was continued alone for two and one-half years, and then was continued for another year with isoniazid 100 mg three times daily. Antituberculosis chemotherapy was discontinued in February, 1953, and has not been given since. During the period of chemotherapy the pulmonary lesion healed; the cavities closed and the sputum became negative. There has been no reactivation.

The urine culture was last positive in May, 1952. The patient has had annual check-ups since his discharge. The last check-up was performed in August, 1964. At that time cystoscopy showed the bladder to be heavily injected, with two large diverticula but no ulceration. Retrograde pyelograms showed pelvocalyceal changes in the right kidney. The left ureter was totally obstructed, permitting no dye to pass into the pelvis, but intravenous pyelography showed a left hydronephrosis and hydroureter, with almost no excretory function in this kidney. The prostrate and seminal vesicles were chronically infected, but there was no evidence of tuberculosis. The urine showed many red and white blood cells and 4 plus albumin, but repeated urine cultures were negative for acid-fast bacilli.

The lesion, when first discovered, was extremely extensive, involving both kidneys, the left ureter, the bladder, the prostate and the seminal vesicles. By present day standards, the patient had inadequate therapy. Nevertheless, as a result of chemotherapy he is living, clinically in fairly good health, able to work, and has remained bacteriologically negative for eleven years after the drugs were stopped. The chronic nontuberculous infections of his genitourinary tract are probably a consequence of the obstruction of his left ureter, which might have been prevented by giving treatment earlier, by giving two-drug treatment from the beginning, or by dilating the left ureter when the stricture was first found. The moderately successful result in this highly unfavorable case shows how very effective drug therapy can be in genitourinary tuberculosis.

SKELETAL TUBERCULOSIS

Like other forms of extrapulmonary tuberculosis, most tuberculosis of bones and joints is traceable to a blood-borne spread of tubercle bacilli which occurs soon after the primary infection. Also like other forms of extrapulmonary tuberculosis, clinical bone and joint lesions may occur within a few months of the initial infection or may appear years later. For many years skeletal lesions developed in about 5 per cent of children with pulmonary primary tuberculosis (12). The percentage of patients with chronic pulmonary tuberculosis who had bone and joint lesions was likewise high, being reported as 3.8 per cent in 1941 (13). However, the virtual eradication of bovine tuberculosis and, more especially, the wide-spread treatment of primary tuberculosis with isoniazid have greatly reduced the incidence of skeletal tuberculosis.

Tuberculosis can involve any bone or joint, but most cases occur in the spine, hip and knee. The bone lesion begins in most cases in the epiphyses. Progression of the caseous process may result in extension into the neighboring soft tissues, with the formation of cold abscesses, or may involve the joint capsule.

Tuberculosis of the spine involves first the body of the vertebra. Progression of the lesion often causes sufficient destruction of one or more vertebral bodies, resulting in collapse of those bodies and kyphosis. Extension of the process into the soft tissues causes the formation of cold abscesses, and these may rupture, forming persistent draining sinuses. Muscle spasm is common in tuberculosis of the spine. The diagnosis should be suspected from the signs and symptoms, and even more from the x-ray evidence of a destructive bone lesion. The finding of a cold abscess is strong evidence of tuberculosis, and the diagnosis is made with certainty by the finding of tubercle bacilli in the discharge from a draining sinus or in the pus from a cold abscess.

Tuberculosis of joints is usually accompanied by a rather severe local pain, which is increased by motion and decreased by immobilization. Pain is due to increased tension in the joint, and to the destructive lesion of the joint surface and nearby bone. There is often swelling about the joint. Muscle spasm is common, and muscle atrophy is likewise common. If untreated, ankylosis of the joint may occur, with the possibility of healing but with the certainty of loss of function; in addition, spontaneous ankylosis is likely to immobilize the involved joint in an unfavorable position.

Successful treatment should heal the disease with a minimum of anatomical deformity and functional loss. This requires both chemotherapy and a measure of rest for the affected parts. Rest for the affected parts should be carried out under the supervision of an orthopedist. The location of the tuberculosis and the extent of the destructive process when treatment is first started will determine the type of rest and its duration. Bed rest, splints, braces, casts and even bony fusion may be required. In general, the more effective the chemotherapy, the shorter the duration of rest and the less stringently it needs to be carried out. Formerly, inactivity in casts was necessary for long periods of time, and surgical fusion was common. Today fusion is only an occasional adjunct to chemotherapy. Chemotherapy alone is successful in curing the disease in the majority of cases, from childhood to old age, so that fusion is usually unnecessary and joint function can be preserved (14) (15) (16).

Chemotherapy should consist of two effective drugs, by preference isoniazid 100 mg three times daily and streptomycin 1 gm daily. Effective chemotherapy stops the growth and multiplication of tubercle bacilli, reduces inflammation and the resulting pain, and cuts short the destruction of bone and joint. Obviously it is of the greatest importance to begin drug treatment early, before much tissue destruction has occurred, for, although some repair can take place, the more destruction that has taken place the greater the loss of function is likely to be. Chemotherapy should be continued for two years or longer. Even in the most advanced cases, prolonged therapy may produce healing, so it is worthwhile to postpone surgical fusion until a long course of drug treatment has been given. Surgical fusion of tuberculous joints is best avoided, if possible, since this inevitably causes permanent functional damage. Spinal fusion is still performed fairly often in the treatment of tuberculous spondylitis, but even here there is a group of physicians who prefer to treat this disease by chemotherapy alone and who claim excellent results (17) (18).

Chemotherapy of primary tuberculosis has greatly reduced the incidence of skeletal tuberculosis. Chemotherapy of skeletal tuberculosis has practically eliminated its mortality and greatly reduced the crippling that used to be so common in this disease.

TUBERCULOSIS OF SEROUS CAVITIES

Tuberculous Pleurisy. This fairly common form of tuberculosis arises usually by extension from a subpleural focus. It may also develop as the result of the direct implantation of tubercle bacilli on the pleura during a hematogenous dissemination. Almost always there is an outpouring of fluid, accompanied by inspiratory pain, fever, and dyspnea. Though a large percentage of so-called "idiopathic effusions" are tuberculous in origin, it is not proper to treat them as such without making every effort to establish an etiologic diagnosis, because in some cases the cause might be a neoplasm or a fungus infection.

A tuberculin test should be done; in tuberculous effusions this is almost always positive. The pleural fluid should be examined and cultured for tubercle bacilli. If the pleural smear is negative, a pleural biopsy should be done. Appropriate studies should be carried out for the detection of cancer and fungus infections. As soon as these tests have been done, if no definite diagnosis has been made, antituberculosis treatment should be started while awaiting the results of the cultures. In itself, tuberculous pleurisy is rather benign; even without treatment the effusion usually absorbs spontaneously. However, without chemotherapy 50 per cent of the patients who have a tuberculous pleurisy with effusion later develop chronic pulmonary tuberculosis (19). Chemotherapy has very little effect on the tuberculous pleurisy with effusion, neither reducing the duration of fever nor speeding the absorption of fluid. The value of effective chemotherapy is that it reduces the later incidence of pulmonary and extrapulmonary tuberculosis to less than 5 per cent (20). Effective chemotherapy consists of treatment with two drugs, one of which should be isoniazid, for a period of two years. A good regimen is isoniazid 100 mg three times daily and PAS 4 gm three times daily. In spite of the apparent benignity of this form of tuberculosis, relapses have occurred in patients who have had a year of treatment, so it is worthwhile to continue chemotherapy for a full two years.

Tuberculous Pericarditis. This is an uncommon but serious form of tuberculosis. Infection of the pericardium may occur by way of the blood stream or by extension from a nearby tuberculous lymph node. The great majority of patients have active tuberculosis elsewhere in the body, and others have evidence of inactive tuberculosis elsewhere. It is exceptional to find pericardial tuberculosis without any evidence of the disease elsewhere in the body, and in these cases it must be presumed that the primary infection was small and healed well. At the time the patient is first seen, the most common symptoms are fever, chest pain, dyspnoea and tachycardia, and the most common signs are enlarged heart, friction rub and pleural effusion. There is often enough pericardial fluid to cause tamponade (21). Before drug treatment, there was a high mortality during the acute phase of the disease, and many others died later as a result of the constrictive pericarditis which often followed; the total mortality was more than 80 per cent (22) (23).

As a result of the reduction in the incidence of pulmonary tuberculosis, and as a result of the drug treatment of primary tuberculosis, the frequency of tuberculous pericarditis has decreased greatly (24). Chemotherapy is very effective, the best combination being streptomycin 1 gm daily and isoniazid 100 mg three times daily. Drugs should be given for at least two years. Steroids are indicated in this condition to diminish the risk of the later development of constrictive pericarditis. Prednisolone may be given for this purpose in doses of 15 or 20 mg three times daily for three or four days; this may then be reduced to 10 mg three times daily, which is continued until the effusion has absorbed, and then tapered off. If constrictive pericarditis develops nevertheless, pericardiectomy must be performed.

Tuberculous Peritonitis. This is usually due to extension of infection from nearby tuberculous lymph nodes, from tuberculous intestinal ulcers, or from infected Fallopian tubes. It may arise also as a result of direct implantation of tubercle bacilli in the course of hematogenous dissemination, but this is less common. In the female, extension from an infected Fallopian tube is by far the commonest route of involvement (25). It may take the form of a plastic peritonitis, with very little fluid, or it may be associated with the outpouring of a large amount of fluid. The plastic form is productive of many adhesions which cause loops of the intestines to mat together, often causing intestinal obstruction. When fluid is present, there is usually fever and abdominal pain. The diagnosis should be considered when there is unexplained fever, weight loss, abdominal pain, tenderness, intestinal obstruction or ascites. It should be strongly suspected when there is evidence of tuberculosis elsewhere in the body, or when the ascitic fluid is rich in protein (3.5 gm or more per 100 ml). A definite diagnosis is made following the finding of tubercle bacilli in the peritoneal fluid, or following peritoneoscopy or laparatomy with the obtaining of material for histological and bacteriological examination (26) (27) (28). Like other forms of extrapulmonary tuberculosis, tuberculous peritonitis is becoming less and less frequent. The treatment consists of two-drug chemotherapy, isoniazid 100 mg three times daily and PAS 4 gm three times daily, or isoniazid 100 mg three times daily and streptomycin 1 gm daily, continued for two years.

TUBERCULOSIS OF LARYNX AND BRONCHI

Tuberculous Laryngitis. Once this was common, serious and difficult to treat, but since the advent of antituberculosis chemotherapy the whole character of this complication has changed markedly for the better. Tuberculous laryngitis causes pain in the throat, hoarseness or even complete aphonia, and pain on swallowing. The disease usually begins with swelling of the mucous membrane in the posterior commissure and the arytenoids. Later the process involves the vocal cords and the epiglottis, and extensive ulceration takes place. Finally, in untreated cases there may be extensive scarring and stenosis of the airway. Treatment without drugs was unsatisfactory. Chemotherapy produces spectacular results, with relief of symptoms in a few days and healing of the lesions in a few weeks. Two-drug therapy is required. The disease heals rapidly, so the duration of treatment is governed by the time required for the management of the pulmonary tuberculosis which practically always accompanies it.

Tuberculous Bronchitis. Tuberculosis of the bronchi is still fairly common when a patient with active pulmonary tuberculosis presents himself for treatment, but is most uncommon as an independent lesion apart from pulmonary disease. It may take the forms of inflammation, granulation or ulceration of the bronchial mucosa. If untreated, bronchial obstruction may occur as a result. Healing is prompt and complete when effective chemotherapy is employed, so that bronchial tuberculosis is seldom of much importance in the medical management of pulmonary tuberculosis. If resectional surgery is performed in the presence of active bronchial tuberculosis, there is considerable danger that the bronchial stump will ulcerate. It is, therefore, important that the patient should receive adequate chemotherapy prior to surgical resection. Since the bronchial lesion usually heals long before the pulmonary disease becomes stable enough for surgery, postoperative ulceration of the bronchial stump is uncommon. It is more common in patients who are receiving retreatment, since their bacilli may be resistant to one or both of the drugs they are receiving, so that their chemotherapy may not really be effective. A good regime consists of isoniazid 100 mg three times daily with either PAS 4 gm three times daily or streptomycin 1 gm daily. If resectional surgery is performed, the drugs should be continued for at least two months postoperatively. In other cases, the duration of treatment is dependent on the need.

TUBERCULOSIS OF THE ALIMENTARY TRACT

Tuberculosis of the Mouth. Tuberculosis sometimes involves the mucous membrane of the mouth and tongue, producing ulcerations which may be shallow or deep. Usually these forms of tuberculosis occur as complications of extensive pulmonary disease. The ulcers of the tongue and oropharynx may be very painful. The diagnosis is made by the finding of tubercle bacilli in the sputum or in smears from the ulcers, and by the demonstration of concomitant pulmonary tuberculosis. Biopsy of the ulcers will make a positive diagnosis but is not desirable because it is likely to make the pain much worse.

Treatment with isoniazid 100 mg three times daily accompanied by streptomycin 1 gm daily or by PAS four gm three times daily, is rapidly effective. On this treatment the pain usually disappears within a few days and the ulcers heal within a few weeks. The duration of treatment depends on the requirements of the pulmonary disease which accompanies the oropharyngeal tuberculosis.

Tuberculosis of the Esophagus and Stomach. These organs are very rarely involved by tuberculosis. The treatment is two-drug therapy, continued as long as needed by the underlying pulmonary disease.

Tuberculosis of the Intestines. Once this was a very common complication of pulmonary tuberculosis. It arises as a result of infection of the intestinal mucosa by tubercle bacilli in swallowed sputum. At first there is infiltration only, but in a short time this is replaced by shallow ulceration. The early lesions are usually to be found in the ileocecal region, but in severe cases ulceration may involve much of the jejunum and ileum, and much of the large bowel as far as the sigmoid colon. The ulcers rarely perforate the intestine, and because they run in a longitudinal direction they rarely cause obstruction. The early symptoms are simply those of chronic disease-weakness, weight loss and fever. As the ulceration becomes more extensive localizing symptoms may appear, such as abdominal cramps and diarrhoea. When these symptoms occur in the presence of active pulmonary tuberculosis, it is safe to make the diagnosis of intestinal tuberculosis and to treat accordingly. The treatment consists of the administration of two antituberculosis drugs in standard doses. The symptoms clear up with great rapidity, and the ulcers heal well. The duration of treatment depends on the underlying pulmonary tuberculosis. Tuberculosis of the intestines was once both a common and a formidable complication of pulmonary tuberculosis, but it has become uncommon and is no longer to be feared.

Tuberculous Ischiorectal Abscess and Fistula-in-ano. These conditions are uncommon complications of pulmonary tuberculosis, though before the days of effective antituberculosis drugs they were quite common. They arise, like intestinal tuberculosis, as a result of infection by tubercle bacilli which are present in swallowed sputum. They require both surgical treatment and antituberculosis drugs. Ischiorectal abscess requires incision and drainage and fistula-in-ano requires excision. In both cases effective antituberculosis therapy should precede and follow surgery, otherwise persistent draining sinuses are likely to develop. The presence of coexisting pulmonary tuberculosis makes it probable that the cause of the local lesion is likewise tuberculosis, and the typical response to drugs makes the diagnosis even more probable. A definite diagnosis can only be made by finding tubercle bacilli in the pus or drainage, or by finding tuberculous granulation tissue in the surgical specimen. Chemotherapy consists of two antituberculosis drugs, given for a period of two years.

TUBERCULOSIS OF LYMPH NODES

Tuberculosis of the regional lymph nodes is an essential part of every primary tuberculous infection. Not only are the regional lymph nodes involved, but there is an early dissemination of tubercle bacilli through the lymph channels and blood stream, so that distant lymph nodes are often involved also. Usually this early infection heals, but sometimes the infection progresses, and sometimes it becomes dormant but becomes reactivated months or years later. Tuberculosis of the lymph nodes usually involves a chain of such nodes rather than a single gland. The nodes tend to caseate, to become matted together, and to enlarge. If untreated they may heal, but on the other hand they may progress, soften, and form one or more draining sinuses.

The great majority of superficial tuberculous lymph nodes occur in the cervical region, and in most cases they are associated with chronic pulmonary tuberculosis. At first the nodes are noticed as enlarged, discrete, painless and nontender. As the disease progresses the swelling increases in size and may become somewhat painful and tender. If further progression occurs, the nodes mat together in a large, irregular mass which liquefies and forms a cold abscess, and which may break through the skin and result in one or more persistent draining sinuses. A definite diagnosis is made by finding tubercle bacilli in the drainage, or in the pus obtained by aspirating an abscess.

Surgical excision is sometimes desirable; it may shorten the duration of the disease, and it may produce a better cosmetic result. Under the protection of the antituberculosis drugs, excision can be carried out without the risk of causing persistent draining sinuses.

Fundamentally, however, treatment with the antituberculosis drugs is the basic treatment. Though isoniazid alone may produce good healing, it is better to give two drugs from the start. Tuberculous lymphadenitis is relatively benign, but because of its tendency to relapse it should be treated for at least two years and often longer (29). The response is likely to be slow. Sinuses heal promptly, but the swollen glands regress very slowly.

Other forms of tuberculosis are now rare. Tuberculosis of the skin, eyes, ears or adrenal glands was never common, and is now seen with the greatest infrequency. When these forms do occur, however, they respond to the same drugs as other forms of tuberculosis.

SUMMARY

Tuberculosis may involve not only the lungs, but any organ and structure in the body. Because of earlier diagnosis and better treatment of primary tuberculosis, all forms of extrapulmonary tuberculosis are diminishing in frequency, and some are quite rare. When they occur, they respond satisfactorily to treatment with the antituberculosis drugs. The same principles apply to the treatment of extrapulmonary as pulmonary tuberculosis—the use of two or more effective drugs, the use of adequate dosages, and the continuation of treatment for not less than two years. The results of such treatment are excellent.

REFERENCES

1. FALK, A., Results of treatment in miliary tuberculosis. *Amer. Rev. Resp. Dis., 91*:6, 1965.

2. MILOCHEVITCH, R.: Les tuberculoses miliaires du poumon. *Rev. Tuberc. (Paris), 27*:600, 1963.

3. RICH, A. R., AND McCORDOCK, H. A.: The pathogenesis of tuberculous meningitis. *Bull. Hopkins Hosp., 52*:5, 1933.

4. WRIGHT, N. L.: Treatment of tuberculous meningitis. *Quart. J. Med., 28*:449, 1959.

5. WASZ-HOCKERT, O., AND DONNER, M.: A follow-up of 103 children recovered from tuberculous meningitis. *Acta Paediat., (Uppsala), suppl., 141*:26, 1963.

6. PERNOD, J., CHAMBATTE, C., BATIME, J., AND KERMAREC, J.: Re-

sultats de la therapeutique de la meningite tuberculeuse de l'adulte. *Rev. Tuberc. (Paris), 26*:205, 1962.

7. WEISS, W., AND FLIPPIN, H. F.: The prognosis of tuberculous meningitis in the isoniazid era. *Amer. J. Med. Sci., 242*:423, 1961.

8. FALK, A.: Tuberculous meningitis in adults with special reference to survival, neurologic residuals, and work status. *Amer. Rev. Resp. Dis., 91*:823, 1965.

9. MEDLAR, E. M.: The significance of tubercle bacilli in the urine. *Urol. Cutan. Rev., 36*:71, 1932.

10. GIRGIS, A. S., AND LATTIMER, J. K.: The chemotherapy of genitourinary tuberculosis with regimens using cycloserine. *J. Urol., 87*:9, 1962.

11. The Present Status of Genitourinary Tuberculosis, A statement of the Committee on Therapy. *Amer. Rev. Resp. Dis., 92*:505, 1965.

12. LINCOLN, E. M., AND SEWELL, E. M.: *Tuberculosis in Children.* New York, McGraw-Hill, 1963.

13. ROSENCRANTZ, E., PISCITELLI, A., AND BOST, F. C.: An analytical study of bone and joint lesions in relation to chronic pulmonary tuberculosis. *J. Bone Joint Surg., 23*:628, 1941.

14. WEBER, R., AND BERLEMON, M.: La tuberculose de la hanche chez l'adulte. *Rev. Chir. Orthop., 46*:504, 1960.

15. McTAMMANY, J. R., MOSER, K. M., AND HOUK, V. N.: Disseminated bone tuberculosis. Review of the literature and presentation of an unusual case. *Amer. Rev. Resp. Dis., 87*:889, 1963.

16. MILKAU, A.: Verlauf und Behandlung der Knochen-und Gelenktuberkulose beim alten Menschen. *Arch. Orthop. Unfall-chir., 55*:36, 1963.

17. KONSTAM, P. G., AND BLESOVSKY, A.: The ambulant treatment of spinal tuberculosis. *Brit. J. Surg., 50*:26, 1962.

18. STEVENSON, F. H., AND MANNING, C. W.: Tuberculosis of the spine treated conservatively with chemotherapy. *Tubercle, 43*:406, 1962.

19. ROPER, W. H., AND WARING, J. J.: Primary serofibrinous pleural effusion in military personnel. *Amer. Rev. Tuberc., 71*:616, 1955.

20. FALK, A., AND STEAD, W. W.: Antimicrobial therapy in the treatment of primary tuberculous pleurisy with effusion; its effect upon the incidence of subsequent tuberculous relapse. *Amer. Rev. Tuberc., 74*:897, 1956.

21. BAUER, H., ROBINS, M., SACHS, R., AND CUMMINGS, M. M.: Tuberculous pericarditis among veterans. *Trans. 15th Conf. Chemotherapy of Tuberculosis*, p. 138, 1956.

22. BOUVRAIN, Y., AND PAGES—DARTEVILLE, S.: The prognosis of peri-carditis. *Sem. Hop. Paris, 31*:831, 1955.

23. SALEM, M. H., AND WILSON, J. R.: Tuberculous pericarditis. *J. Int. Coll. Surg., 33*:535, 1960.

24. SCHEPERO, G. W. H.: Tuberculous pericarditis. *Amer. J. Cardiol., 9*:248, 1962.

25. KARDOS, F., AND SZOLGA, I.: Peritonealtuberkulose und weibliche Genitaltuberkulose. *Acta Chir. Acad. Sci. Hung., 4*:221, 1963.

26. HYMAN, S., VILLA, F., ALVAREZ, S., AND STEIGMANN, E.: The enigma of tuberculous peritonitis. *Gastroenterology, 42*:1, 1962.

27. GIRARD, M., PLANCHU, M., AND MICHEL, J.: Considerations sur le traitement actual des peritonitis tuberculeuses de l'adulte Arch. Mal. Appar. Dig., *49*:770, 1960.

28. HUGHES, H. J., CARR, D. T., AND GERACI, J. E.: Tuberculous peri-tonitis. *Dis. Chest., 38*:42, 1960.

29. FRIEDMAN, O. H., AND SELIKOFF, I. J.: The chemotherapy of per-ipheral tuberculous lymphadenitis. *J. Mt. Sinai Hospital, N. Y., 23*:529, 1956.

Chapter X

RELAPSE DURING AND AFTER CHEMOTHERAPY

RELAPSE IS DEFINED as deterioration in the course of tuberculosis after initial improvement and conversion of sputum. The deterioration may be bacteriological, radiological or clinical, or any combination of these. The most common and least significant relapses are those which are bacteriological alone.

The relapse rate is influenced by many factors. Patients with extensive pulmonary disease at the beginning of therapy are more likely to relapse than others with less extensive disease, and those with large cavities are more likely to relapse than similar patients with smaller cavities or no cavities. Young patients tend to have less relapses than older ones. Emotional instability, alcoholism and lack of cooperation increase the risk of relapse. Tuberculosis of recent onset not only responds better to chemotherapy than more established disease, but is attended by a smaller risk of relapse. The emergence of drug-resistant tubercle bacilli greatly increases the probability of relapse. Drug toxicity and hypersensitivity may require interruption of treatment and thus favor relapse. Ineffective drug management often results in relapse, and there are many ways in which drug management may be ineffective — there may be a poor choice of drugs, the dosage may be too small, the drugs may not be given (or taken) frequently enough, or the duration of treatment may be too short. Of all the factors that influence the development of relapse, the most important are the extent and cavitary nature of the original tuberculous lesion and the adequacy of chemotherapy (1) (2). As has been stated earlier, adequate drug treatment usually requires the use of two drugs to which the tubercle bacilli are susceptible, given in adequate doses, without interruption, and in most cases for not less than two years.

Because of the many factors which influence the relapse rate, different investigators report widely differing relapse rates. However, everyone agrees that effective chemotherapy has greatly reduced the frequency of relapse. In Sweden, the incidence of relapse was 20.6 per cent in 1952-1955 and 6.4 per cent in 1956-1958 (3). In an American Veterans Administration hospital, the frequency of relapse in those who had received two-drug therapy for two years or more was 4 per cent in 1955-1956 (2), and in an American Army hospital it was only 0.9 per cent (4).

Though the frequency of relapse has been greatly reduced by chemotherapy, the pattern of relapse has not changed much. Most relapses still occur in the first year or eighteen months of therapy. It has been reported that 60 per cent of relapses occur in the first year, 85 per cent in the first two years, and the remaining 15 per cent are scattered over the next two or three years (5). A few relapses occur shortly after chemotherapy has been discontinued. These might be prevented or postponed by prolonged chemotherapy, and so might relapses due to exogenous reinfection, but otherwise there is little to be gained by continuing chemotherapy longer than two years in the hope of avoiding relapses.

The source of relapse is the tuberculous cavity in almost all cases. Therefore it is worthwhile at this point to review the effect of anti-tuberculosis drugs both on tubercle bacilli and on the tuberculous cavity.

The drugs act on actively multiplying tubercle bacilli, and are relatively ineffective against bacilli in the resting state. Therefore, if effective chemotherapy is given to a patient who has a cavity with many millions of tubercle bacilli, most of the bacilli will be suppressed, since they are multiplying and are susceptible to one or both of the drugs which are being used. The organisms which are multiplying but are resistant to both drugs will continue to multiply, so that eventually a resistant bacterial population will exist. Inadequate treatment hastens this unfortunate chain of events—treatment with drugs which are taken irregularly or for too short a period of time, and especially treatment with two drugs to one of which the bacilli are already resistant. Inadequate treatment, leading to the early development of drug-resistant strains of bacilli, is a frequent cause of relapse. The organisms which are in a resting state will not be affected by the drugs, whether they are susceptible or resistant; they are not multiplying but are capable of persisting, and in time they may resume the ability of multiplying and may then produce a relapse.

This phenomenon of bacterial persistence in spite of adequate chemotherapy has not been as well understood as the development of drug resistance, but it may sometimes cause relapse. It explains the sometimes surprising finding that, after a year or more of effective drug treatment there is a bacteriological relapse, and the bacteria which reappear are drug-susceptible. Another explanation for relapse resulting from drug-susceptible bacilli is the excavation of a previously closed, non-cavitary lesion, with the freeing of large numbers of susceptible bacilli into the bronchial tree; but this is an uncommon event.

When antituberculosis drugs are given to a patient with a tuberculous cavity, the broncho-cavitary junction heals and the bronchus remains open, while the cavity may close with inspissation of the contained necrotic material. The tubercle bacilli in the inspissated material may persist in small numbers for a considerable period of time. Sometimes liquefaction occurs, and the softened necrotic material passes through the open bronchus and is expectorated, bearing with it a few tubercle bacilli. If the sputum is examined at this time it would be positive, and the patient would be said to have a bacteriologic relapse. However, the number of bacilli is small, the sputum remains positive for only a short time, and there is no spread of disease. Sometimes the cavity does not close with inspissation, especially if it has existed for some months and has a thick wall. Such a cavity may eventually heal while remaining open, the inner wall becoming clean and covered with a hyaline membrane or even with epithelium which grows in from the broncho-cavitary junction. If this "open-healing" is not complete, though, the inner wall may continue to have necrotic material and this necrotic material may contain large numbers of viable tubercle bacilli. These bacilli can grow readily, and if aspirated into the bronchial tree they are capable of causing a spread of disease, thus causing both a bacteriologic and radiologic relapse.

There is still another route by which a relapse can occur, and this is by exogenous reinfection. Exogenous reinfection is certainly possible. It can be established in experimental animals; when they have recovered from active tuberculosis as a result of chemotherapy, they can be reinfected by causing them to inhale droplets containing tubercle bacilli. It can be proven to exist in man, too. Patients who recovered from pulmonary tuberculosis in the pre-chemotherapy era have developed new lesions in recent years, and these lesions have yielded tubercle bacilli resistant to one or more antituberculosis drugs before the patient received any chemotherapy, indicating an infection with a new strain of tubercle bacilli. However, when a patient has recovered from pulmonary tuberculosis, his immunity is likely to be quite high, so that he is not likely to become reinfected from without. It is generally believed that exogenous reinfection is an uncommon occurrence.

The fate of patients who suffer relapses is not necessarily bad. Those whose relapse is only bacteriological, without any clinical evidence of renewed activity and without any radiological evidence of spread, fare particularly well; on continued chemotherapy their sputum usually becomes negative again and they have no further difficulty. Even those who have relapses which are demonstrable clinically and radiologically usually recover. It is necessary to change the drug therapy, and in many cases resectional surgery is strongly indicated. Since the major source of relapse is the residual cavity, an important part of the attack on the relapse should be the resection of the cavity. About three quarters of all patients who have relapses eventually recover.

SUMMARY

A relapse is a deterioration of the pulmonary tuberculosis after initial improvement. The deterioration may be clinical, bacteriological or radiological or a combination of these. Following adequate chemotherapy, the incidence of relapse has been greatly reduced, and is now about 5 per cent. Most relapses occur within two years of the beginning of treatment. Following relapse, it is necessary to change the drug therapy so that two effective drugs are always being used. The source of most relapses is the residual cavity, and the treatment of most relapses includes resection of the residual cavity. About three quarters of all patients who have relapses eventually recover.

REFERENCES

1. RIGGINS, H. M.: Relapse after medical treatment of pulmonary tuberculosis: host, bacterial, drug, and medical factors. *Bull. Int. Un. Tuberc., 30*:412, 1960.

2. PHILLIPS, S.: Relapse in treated cases of pulmonary tuberculosis. *Amer. Rev. Resp. Dis., 90*:61, 1964.

3. LARMOLA, E.: On the incidence of relapses in pulmonary tuberculosis. *Acta. Tuberc., Scand., 41*:92, 1962.

4. WIER, J. A., DUNNINGTON, W. G., AND TEMPEL, C. W.: Progress in the Army's tuberculosis program. *Milit. Med., 126*:589, 1961.

5. MIDDLEBROOK, G., STEELE, J. D.,AUERBACH, O., EDWARDS, F. R., EPSTEIN, I., FROMAN, S., RALEIGH, J. W., ROBSON, J. M., AND STEENKEN, W.: The problem of relapse of tuberculous lesions under chemotherapy and following treatment. *Amer. Rev. Resp. Dis., 80, Part 2*:47, 1959.

Chapter XI

TUBERCULOSIS IN CHILDREN

TUBERCULOSIS IN CHILDREN is in many ways different from tuberculosis in adults (1). There are differences in duration, extent and destructiveness of the disease, and consequently there are differences in prognosis, management and drug treatment. Tuberculosis in children is usually of recent origin, and in most cases the lesions to be treated are small in extent, primary or early post-primary in character, and involve little tissue destruction. Extrapulmonary tuberculosis is more common in children than in adults. Children are less likely to develop toxic reactions to the antituberculosis drugs than are adults even when large doses are used. The development of bacillary strains resistant to the antituberculosis drugs is uncommon in children, because cavitary disease sheltering large populations of rapidly-growing tubercle bacilli is uncommon in children. Treatment failure is uncommon in children for this reason, unless treatment is delayed until the child is moribund.

As in adult tuberculosis, two-drug therapy is more effective than single-drug therapy. Isoniazid is adequate by itself for prophylaxis or for therapy of primary tuberculosis which is producing no signs or symptoms; but for the treatment of established tuberculosis in children, therapy with two drugs is preferred. Isoniazid accompanied by daily streptomycin is the most effective combination in the treatment of tuberculosis in children, as it is in adults, and isoniazid and PAS is another good combination. The dosage of isoniazid recommended is 10 mg per kg body weight daily, given in two or three divided doses, but larger doses may be given when the disease threatens life. It is seldom necessary to give more than 400 mg daily. Streptomycin is given in doses ranging from 0.3 gm daily for children who weigh less than 5 kg to 1 gm daily for children who weigh 40 kg or more (1). PAS is given in doses of about 0.2 gm per kg, with slightly larger doses per kg being given to smaller children.

Toxic reactions to isoniazid are almost unknown in children. Streptomycin causes a number of toxic manifestations in children, though toxicity is less common and less severe than in adults. Hearing loss is infrequent, but vestibular damage is common and may be severe. Itchy skin eruptions are common, and rarely exfoliative dermatitis may occur; the latter requires immediate discontinuation of streptomycin. PAS causes both toxic and allergic manifestations. Toxic reactions — anorexia, nausea, vomiting and diarrhoea — are common, and may be severe enough to require the drug to be stopped. Allergic manifestations, too, are fairly common, usually in the form of fever, skin rashes and eosinophilia. Febrile reactions require discontinuation of the drug; desensitization is usually possible, and must be accomplished if the drug is to be used again.

The secondary drugs are needed much less frequently in children than in adults. Secondary drugs are needed when the use of the primary drugs is not feasible because of toxicity, or when the primary drugs are not effective because the tubercle bacilli are resistant to them. We have seen that toxicity is less frequent in children than in adults, and the development of resistant bacilli is very much less frequent. Adequate treatment with the primary drugs is successful in children in the great majority of cases. Nevertheless, the secondary drugs are occasionally needed, and any of the drugs used for adults may be used in the treatment of children.

Pyrazinamide may be used in doses of 30 mg per kg body weight daily, in two or three divided doses, not to exceed a total dosage of 1.5 gm daily. It occasionally causes a toxic hepatitis, and less commonly it may produce an elevation of the serum uric acid. Ethionamide is effective in dosages of 500 mg daily in adults, and in proportionately lower dosages in children. It often produces nausea and anorexia, and occasionally causes a toxic hepatitis. Cycloserine is a highly effective drug, often rendering the sputum negative and promoting clinical improvement when other drugs have failed. It is not widely used because of its neurotoxicity, since in some cases it causes headache, drowsiness, convulsions and even psychoses. When pyridoxine is given with cycloserine, the frequency of convulsions is greatly reduced, but psychosis still occurs. Even though psychosis is a rare complication and usually a transient one, its occurrence limits the use of this otherwise valuable drug. The dose is 10 mg per kg body weight. Viomycin, in doses of 30 mg per kg body weight, is also an effective drug. It should be given twice weekly. Its toxicity is similar to that of streptomycin — damage to hearing or to vestibular function is fairly common, and renal irritation, with the occurrence of albumin and casts in the urine, is also fairly common. The secondary drugs are needed much less frequently in children than in adults, but a number of useful drugs are available if needed.

Pulmonary tuberculosis in children may be either primary or reinfection type. Most primary pulmonary tuberculosis heals spontaneously, but it is worth treating aggressively because of the serious complications (such as miliary and meningeal tuberculosis), which may occur during the period immediately after primary infection as a result of blood-stream dissemination. Treatment of primary pulmonary tuberculosis will also prevent most extrapulmonary tuberculosis and most reinfection-type pulmonary tuberculosis (2). Adequate chemotherapy of asymptomatic pulmonary primary tuberculosis requires isoniazid only. This drug, in doses of 10 mg per kg body weight for a period of one year, is almost always sufficient to prevent complications (1) (3).

Progressive primary pulmonary tuberculosis is uncommon, but is serious, since it usually results in cavitation, dissemination of tu bercle bacilli throughout the lungs, and the development of areas of tuberculous bronchopneumonia. Such patients need treatment with two drugs as soon as the diagnosis is made. Usually isoniazid 10 mg per kg and PAS 0.2 gm per kg are adequate. However, if the disease is acute or extensive or the patient is in poor condition, it may be desirable to give streptomycin 20 mg per kg daily for several months in place of PAS; after the patient seems definitely on the road to recovery, streptomycin may be discontinued and PAS substituted. Treatment should be continued for eighteen to twenty-four months. In refractory cases, drug treatment should be maintained for six months after the sputum or gastric contents have become negative and all evidence of cavitation has disappeared from view on the chest x rays. Since progressive primary pulmonary tuberculosis often involves cavitation and the production of large numbers of tubercle bacilli, children with this type of tuberculosis are infectious and must be isolated. This is an entirely different situation from the usual forms of primary tuberculosis in children, in which excretion of tubercle bacilli is minimal or absent and infectiousness does not exist.

Primary extrapulmonary tuberculosis is uncommon in children as in adults. The prognosis is better than in pulmonary disease, because blood-stream dissemination and progressive local disease are both rare. Primary extrapulmonary tuberculosis involves, of course, both a local lesion at the portal of entry and involvement of the draining lymph nodes. Both portions of the primary complex tend to heal spontaneously. Chemotherapy is desirable, however, to minimize scarring, heal draining sinuses when they occur, and shorten the course of the disease. The regimen of isoniazid 10 mg per kg body weight and PAS 0.2 gram per kg daily in divided doses is effective.

Chronic pulmonary tuberculosis or reinfection tuberculosis is not frequent in children, but has increased in frequency in adolescents in the past few years. This disease is usually localized in the lungs, and tends not to spread by way of the blood-stream or lymphatics. As in adult tuberculosis, chronic pulmonary tuberculosis in children begins as a microscopic area of tuberculous pneumonia. The bacilli multiply in this focus, the lesion liquefies, and the disease extends both concentrically and by spread through the bronchi. Cavity formation is common. Spontaneous healing is similar in children and adults. Non-cavitary lesions heal by resolution, encapsulation, fibrosis and calcification, though extensive fibrosis is rare in children. Cavities heal by inspissation of their contents or by calcification, with bronchial closure. Following chemotherapy there is a new form of healing. The bronchocavitary junction heals and becomes covered with epithelium, and thereafter the cavity remains open, but may heal by the death of the tubercle bacilli and the growth of epithelium from the bronchcavitary junction into the cavity. This open healing ends with the formation of a clean uninfected cavity, covered with epithelium and free of tubercle bacilli (4) (5).

As in adults, good treatment of chronic pulmonary tuberculosis in children requires that treatment with two drugs, should be started as early as possible, and should be continued for a long time. The basic drugs are almost always satisfactory, as acquired drug resistance is uncommon in children. It is necessary to perform drug susceptibility tests on the patient's tubercle bacilli, because children may be infected by adults whose tubercle bacilli have become resistant to one or another of the basic drugs; if this proves to be true, secondary drugs should be used. In any case, two drugs known to be effective should be given, and treatment should be continued for eighteen months to two years. Adolescent girls are especially vulnerable to tuberculosis, and therefore require even more prolonged treatment. If menstruation begins before or during the planned course of chemotherapy for tuberculosis, drug treatment should be extended for two years after menarche.

Acute miliary tuberculosis is more common in children than in adults, and is most frequent in infants and young children. It occurs typically within a few months after primary infection. Tubercles may be found disseminated throughout the body. The children are acutely ill, and if effective drugs are not given the disease tends to progress. Untreated miliary tuberculosis in children usually ends in death, either from progressive disease or from meningitis. Chemotherapy has reduced the mortality almost to nothing, but since tubercles are widely disseminated and the bacilli may persist for a long time, drug therapy should be started early and continued for at least two years. Two-drug therapy is necessary for good results, and the best results are obtained with streptomycin and isoniazid. An effective regime is streptomycin 1 gm daily and isoniazid 20 mg per kg body weight, continued until the temperature has returned to normal. After that isoniazid should be continued in full doses for another three months, but the frequency of streptomycin may be diminished to twice weekly. Thereafter, the dosage of isoniazid may be reduced to 10 mg per kg body weight daily, PAS 0.2 gm per kg body weight may be substituted for streptomycin, and this combination should be continued until the patient has had two years of effective treatment (6). The corticosteroid hormones need not be used routinely, but in children who are acutely ill the use of the steroids may cause a rapid reduction in fever and a rapid improvement in well-being.

Tuberculous meningitis in children is a rapidly progressive disease which is always fatal unless effective chemotherapy is given. Early diagnosis and treatment are imperative if brain damage is to be prevented. The pathogenesis of this complication is the same in children as in adults. The onset is sudden in a large percentage of young children, with fever and convulsions. In others the onset is gradual, beginning with low-grade fever, vomiting and apathy. The symptoms progress, increasing drowsiness appearing, as well as a positive Kernig sign, absent abdominal reflexes and increased deep reflexes. Finally coma develops, and death follows in a few days. When the diagnosis is suspected on clinical grounds, a positive tuberculin reaction and x-ray evidence of primary tuberculosis strengthen the suspicion. The cerebrospinal fluid typically is clear, with a cell count of 10 to 300 per cu mm. The predominant cell is the lymphocyte. The protein content of the cerebrospinal fluid is elevated and may be very high while the sugar content is reduced. The finding of tubercle bacilli in the fluid makes the diagnosis absolutely certain.

The prognosis is good if drug treatment is started early in the course of the complication, and if it is continued in adequate doses for two years or more. If effective treatment is started late the patient will usually recover but there will be considerable permanent neurological damage, and this may be extensive enough to be disabling (7). Treatment is similar to that of miliary tuberculosis, beginning with large doses of isoniazid and streptomycin, reducing the dosage after two months and later substituting PAS for streptomycin. A recommended regime is isoniazid 20 mg per kg accompanied by streptomycin 1 gm daily for two months, then reducing the isoniazid to 10 mg per kg and the streptomycin to 1 gm twice weekly. After six months, streptomycin may be discontinued and PAS substituted in doses of 0.2 gm per kg and this isoniazid-PAS regime should be continued until the patient has received at least two years of chemotherapy.

Genitourinary tuberculosis is a complication of diminishing frequency. The most common and serious form is renal tuberculosis, from which a descending infection can involve the lower urinary tract. Recommended treatment consists of the three basic drugs — isoniazid 10 mg per kg daily, PAS 0.2 gm per kg daily, and streptomycin 20 mg per kg twice weekly. Streptomycin is given for six months if the urogram is normal, but for eighteen months if the urogram is abnormal; isoniazid and PAS are given for eighteen months in either situation (8). Genital tuberculosis responds well to treatment with two drugs, but early diagnosis and treatment is important. Tuberculous salpingitis and tuberculous epididymitis heal well, but a large percentage of children who have recovered from these complications remain sterile.

Skeletal tuberculosis is an early complication, occurring usually within six months of the primary infection. Any bone in the body may be involved, but, in children, the sites most frequently affected are the spine and the bones of the hands and feet. Any joint in the body may be involved, but the joints which most frequently become tuberculous are the hip and knee. The principles of diagnosis and treatment are much the same as in adults. The key to successful treatment is early and adequate chemotherapy combined with immobilization of the affected parts in the optimum position. Immobilization may be accomplished by splints, casts or braces, or by bed rest, and is almost always temporary. Permanent immobilization by surgical fusion is rarely necessary, since chemotherapy is adequate by itself to heal the tuberculous process in the great majority of cases. Effective chemotherapy requires two drugs to be given until the lesion is stable by x ray and until all evidence of active tuberculosis has come to an end, and for six months thereafter. This means that in most cases drugs must be given for eighteen months or longer. Isoniazid 10 mg per kg with PAS 0.2 gm per kg is a satisfactory combination.

Tuberculous pleurisy is still a fairly common complication of primary tuberculosis in children. It is an early complication, developing within six months of the primary infection in most cases. The prognosis of tuberculous pleurisy is much better in children than in adults; pulmonary tuberculosis seldom develops later in children who have recovered from tuberculous pleurisy. The treatment consists of isoniazid 10 mg per kg and PAS 0.2 gm per kg daily, given for one year or more.

Tuberculous pericarditis and tuberculous peritonitis should receive the same treatment as tuberculous pleurisy, though it may be desirable to continue therapy for a longer time.

Tuberculous laryngitis and bronchitis are rarely seen except as complications of chronic pulmonary or extrapulmonary tuberculosis.

They heal well under the influence of chemotherapy. Their treatment is the treatment of the underlying disease.

Intestinal tuberculosis is fairly common in older children as a complication of chronic pulmonary tuberculosis. Ulcers develop in the ileo-cecal region, and if the disease is more severe, ulcers may be found also in the jejunum, the ascending and even the transverse colon. This complication responds rapidly to treatment with any of the antituberculosis drugs. The treatment is that of the underlying pulmonary disease.

Tuberculous lymphadenitis occurs as part of the primary complex. More common and more important is the lymphadenitis which may occur as a result of the post-primary dissemination. These are found most commonly in the neck. Usually groups of nodes are involved, rather than one node. The pathology has been described in the chapter on Extrapulmonary Tuberculosis. The treatment consists of isoniazid 10 mg per kg and PAS 0.2 gm per kg. The drugs should be continued for one to two years, or even longer; it should be continued as long as there in inflammation, tenderness or discharge, and for six months longer.

SUMMARY

1. Tuberculosis in children is different from tuberculosis in adults. There are differences in duration, extent and destructiveness of the disease.
2. The same drugs are used for children as for adults, though in smaller doses. However, children are less likely to develop toxic reactions to the antituberculosis drugs, and the development of bacillary strains resistant to these drugs is uncommon in children.
3. As in adult tuberculosis, effective therapy requires two drugs, administered for a long time.
4. Primary tuberculosis should be treated, though usually it heals spontaneously. Chemotherapy of primary tuberculosis prevents miliary and meningeal tuberculosis and extrapulmonary tuberculosis.
5. Chronic pulmonary tuberculosis and extrapulmonary tuberculosis require treatment with two drugs (three drugs are recom-

mended for most cases of genitourinary tuberculosis) for eighteen months or longer.

6. Treatment failure is uncommon in children.

REFERENCES

1. LINCOLN, E. M., AND SEWELL, E. M.: *Tuberculosis in Children.* New York, McGraw-Hill, 1963.
2. LINCOLN, E. M.: The effect of antimicrobial therapy on the prognosis of primary tuberculosis in children. *Amer. Rev. Tuberc., 69*:682, 1954.
3. LOTTE, A., NOUFFLARD, H., DEBRE, R., AND BRISSAUD, H. E.: The treatment of primary tuberculosis in childhood. *Pediatrics, 26*: 641, 1960.
4. AUERBACH, O., KATZ, H. L., AND SMALL, M. J.: The effect of streptomycin therapy on the bronchocavitary junction and its relation to cavity healing. *Amer. Rev. Tuberc., 67*:173, 1953.
5. LINCOLN, E. M., GILBERT, L., AND MORALES, S. M.: Chronic pulmonary tuberculosis with known previous primary tuberculosis. *Dis. Chest, 38*:473, 1960.
6. LINCOLN, E. M., AND HOULD, F.: Results of specific treatment of miliary tuberculosis in children. *New Eng. J. Med., 261*:113, 1959.
7. WASZ-HOCKERT, O., AND DONNER, M.: A follow-up of 103 children recovered from tuberculous meningitis. *Acta Paediat. (Uppsala), suppl., 141*:26, 1963.
8. LATTIMER, J. K., AND BOYES, T.: Renal tuberculosis in children. *Pediatrics, 22*.1193, 1958.

Chapter XII

DISEASE CAUSED BY UNCLASSIFIED MYCOBACTERIA

IT HAS BEEN KNOWN for more than three decades that pulmonary disease in human beings is occasionally due to acid-fast bacilli which are different from mammalian tubercle bacilli (1). There were only sporadic cases recognized at first (2), but the number of cases reported has increased considerably in the last ten years. These bacilli have been called "atypical" and "anonymous," but in 1961, the Committee on Diagnostic Standards of the American Thoracic Society designated them "unclassified mycobacteria."

Runyon (3) has proposed a classification of these organisms based on pigment formation and growth characteristics. Groups within this classification are not entirely homogeneous; each group contains more than one strain. The classification is as follows.

GROUP I — PHOTOCHROMOGENS. Colonies develop a yellow pigment if exposed to light during the period of active growth. Bacilli grow at about the same rate as ordinary tubercle bacilli, and, grow equally well at 20° C or at 37° C. Catalase activity is usually strongly positive. M. kansasii is a Group I organism.

GROUP II — SCOTOCHROMOGENS. Colonies develop pigment even when growth takes place entirely in the dark. The color is yellow or orange if these organisms grow in the dark, and reddish if they are exposed to light. Catalase activity is strongly positive.

GROUP III — NONPHOTOCHROMOGENS. These organisms show little or no pigment formation, whether they grow in light or darkness. Growth occurs at about the same rate as in the case of tubercle bacilli. Most Group III organisms are strongly catalase-positive, but some are

weakly positive. The Battey bacillus is the most common organism in Group III.

Group IV — Rapid Growers. Most Group IV bacilli grow
rapidly, colonies appearing in three or four days, and
most produce no pigment. Growth occurs equally well
at 20° C and at 37° C. Typical bacteria of this group
are M. balnei and M. fortuitum.

In some areas of the United States, infections with unclassified
mycobacteria are very common. For instance, in southern Georgia
and northern Florida more than half of all adults have been infected with the Battey bacillus, as shown by a strongly positive reaction to tuberculin made from this organism. In this area, the
Battey bacillus can be recovered from the sputum of 14 per cent of
healthy adults (4). This finding does not necessarily mean clinical
disease, of course; most of these people are free of symptoms of disease
and have perfectly normal chest x rays. Still, these findings are an
indication of widespread infection. Similarly, in parts of Texas and
the Midwest infection with M. kansasii is commoner than infection
with tubercle bacilli. These two bacilli — the Battey bacillus and
M. kansasii — cause the majority of infections due to unclassified
mycobacteria.

There are several possible explanations for the apparent increase
in the number of cases of disease due to unclassified mycobacteria.
There may, of course, be a real though unexplained increase. Another
possibility is that unclassified mycobacteria are actually mutants of
the tubercle bacillus, caused by antituberculosis chemotherapy (5).
This is not likely to be the whole explanation, since most of the
unclassified mycobacteria were recognized before the days of chemotherapy; if they are to be regarded as mutants, it must be postulated
that not only chemotherapeutic drugs but other agents must be able
to cause the same mutations. The most reasonable possibility is that
as the number of cases of true tuberculosis has diminished and bacteriological techniques have improved, cases of disease due to unclassified mycobacteria are much less likely to be mistaken for tuberculosis. It is probable that formerly many of these cases were incorrectly
diagnosed and treated as tuberculosis.

Clinical disease can be caused by M. kansasii (Group I), the

Battey bacillus (Group III), and M. fortuitum (Group IV). The Group II organisms have not been shown to be pathogenic for either laboratory animals or man. Disease due to unclassified mycobacteria can only be distinguished from tuberculosis by careful bacteriological examination. The clinical findings, the x-ray appearance, and even the pathological findings of resected specimens, are entirely compatible with classical tuberculosis. The patients complain of weakness, weight loss, cough, expectoration, hemoptysis, fever, fatigue, night sweats and the other symptoms of tuberculosis. The x rays show shadows indistinguishable from those of tuberculosis, including nodules, exudative lesions, densely scarred lesions and cavities. The pathological appearance of the lesions is likewise indistinguishable from that of tuberculosis (6); the lesions are chronic granulomata, with tubercles and giant cells of the Langhans type. There is nothing in the symptoms, x-ray appearance, or pathological findings which will permit a differential diagnosis to be made between disease due to tubercle bacilli and disease due to unclassified mycobacteria.

Since all other studies fail to differentiate between pulmonary tuberculosis and disease due to unclassified mycobacteria, this differentiation must be made by bacteriologic studies. On microscopic examination, tubercle bacilli and unclassified mycobacteria look identical, but in cultural characteristics and in reaction to biochemical tests there are differences. These differences are in rate of growth, optimum temperature for growth, development of pigment in the dark and on exposure to light, and in degree of catalase and niacin activity. They suffice in most cases to differentiate tubercle bacilli from unclassified mycobacteria and to establish which strain of mycobacteria is the causative agent in a given case.

Even the finding of unclassified mycobacteria in the sputum does not necessarily prove that it is the cause of disease. Often their presence has no clinical significance. Some may be present as saprophytes. The Battey bacillus, which is certainly capable of causing progressive pulmonary disease in human beings, is not always pathogenic; it is often present in the sputum of people who are in good health clinically and whose chest x rays are perfectly normal. In order to make the diagnosis of disease due to unclassified mycobacteria with any confidence, the following conditions must be met.

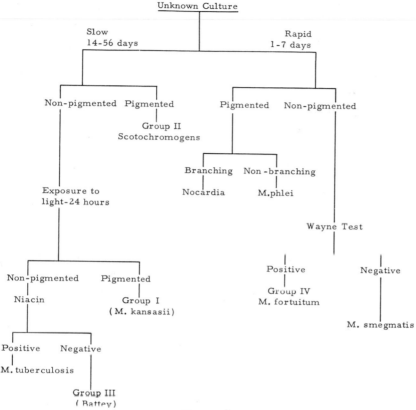

TABLE I

DIFFERENTIATION OF MYCOBACTERIA

1. There must be clinical disease.
2. There must be parenchymal pulmonary disease demonstrable by x ray, or demonstrable glandular disease.
3. Unclassified mycobacteria must be present repeatedly in the sputum or glandular discharge.
4. No other bacteria must be found which could account for the disease.
5. Tissue, if available for examination, must show lesions compatible with disease due to mycobacteria.

There are credible reports of cases in which both the tubercle bacilli and unclassified mycobacteria have been recovered repeatedly from the sputum. In these cases it is likely that two diseases exist, both pulmonary tuberculosis and disease due to unclassified mycobacteria, and that both diseases must be treated.

The epidemiology of the unclassified mycobacteria is still not well understood. Disease due to M. kansasii is widely distributed through the country, though it is most common in Texas and the central states. Both hypersensitivity to the Battey bacillus and disease due to the Battey bacillus are most common in the southeastern states. Disease due to Group IV organisms is uncommon, but cases are reported from widely separated areas. The unusual geographical distribution of these diseases and of skin hypersensitivity to them suggests that some unclassified mycobacteria may be able to survive outside the human host and may even be free-living (7), and, in fact, some of these organisms have been found in soil and water. There is also the possibility that certain people may be healthy "carriers;" this possibility is supported by the fact that many people in certain districts in Georgia have Battey bacilli in their throats and in their sputum, though they are perfectly well clinically and have normal chest x rays.

It is also possible that there may be an animal reservoir of these mycobacteria, and fowl, cats, rats and mice have been considered as potential sources of infection for human beings. The mechanism by which human beings become infected is unknown. Up to the present there have been no confirmed reports of disease due to unclassified mycobacteria in a husband and wife or in two members of the same family, and no human case of this disease has been traced to another case.

Cross sensitization occurs between the various unclassified mycobacteria and tubercle bacilli. Patients with pulmonary disease due to Battey bacilli, for instance, generally have a much stronger reaction to tuberculin prepared from Battey bacilli than to standard tuberculin, but they almost always have a small reaction to standard tuberculin as well. The importance of these cross reactions is unknown.

Two characteristics of the unclassified mycobacteria influence the therapy of the disease they cause. The first is their relative lack of virulence for man. Certainly M. kansasii, the Battey bacillus, and even some Group IV mycobacteria are capable of causing progressive and even fatal disease in man; yet, in general, the disease due to these organisms is more indolent, and the patient is not as severely ill as if he had classical tuberculosis. The second is the fact that the unclassified mycobacteria are usually resistant to many of the antituberculosis drugs even before drug treatment is started.

Group I organisms are usually resistant to streptomycin, isoniazid and PAS, wholly or in part. Most strains are susceptible to cycloserine and ethionamide. Group II organisms have a similar pattern of resistance to drugs, but this is not very important since they are almost avirulent for laboratory animals and man. Group III mycobacteria are usually resistant to all the available drugs. Group IV organisms are likewise highly resistant to drugs in many cases.

Since there is a good deal of variation in the drug-susceptibility patterns of different strains of mycobacteria even within the same group, it is important to determine the susceptibility of each infecting mycobacterium to the entire gamut of the antituberculosis drugs, and to other antibiotics as well, and to use those drugs which seem likely to be most effective on the basis of the susceptibility tests. The basic principles of chemotherapy are the same as for tuberculosis — all patients with active disease should receive drugs, two or more effective drugs should be used concurrently, isoniazid may be effective even if laboratory tests indicate that resistance exists, and drug treatment should be continued without interruption for at least two years and usually longer. When isoniazid is used in spite of a laboratory finding of resistance, it should be administered in doses of 200 mg three times daily, along with pyridoxine to prevent the development of neuritis.

If the principles of drug treatment are no different than in the case of tuberculosis, the results are not as good because the unclassified mycobacteria are usually resistant to many of the drugs from the start. Patients with Group I infections usually fare better than those with infections caused by other unclassified mycobacteria because the degree of initial drug resistance is less; sputum can usually be converted to negative by drugs alone, and cavity closure occurs in a fair percentage (8). The results in Group III and Group IV infections are not quite as good, because of a higher degree of drug resistance at the start of treatment, but even in these cases sputum conversion occurs not infrequently and cavity closure takes place now and then. Since it is not possible to predict the drug-susceptibility pattern of any given strain of bacilli, a good plan is to start the treatment of a new case with three-drug therapy (isoniazid 200 mg three times daily, streptomycin 1 gm daily, and PAS 4 gm three times daily) while awaiting the susceptibility reports from the laboratory (9). When these reports are available, a more intelligent choice of drugs can be made, using two drugs to which the greatest susceptibility exists, and remembering that isoniazid is often effective in patients even when *in vitro* resistance exists. It is also desirable to use first-line drugs in preference to secondary drugs unless the susceptibility tests indicate a high degree of resistance to the former.

As an example, a case of Group I pulmonary infection (M. kansasii) is started on therapy with isoniazid, streptomycin and PAS. Later the laboratory tests show a high degree of resistance to isoniazid and PAS, a low degree of resistance to streptomycin and viomycin, and complete susceptibility to cycloserine and ethionamide. Though laboratory tests of susceptibility to pyrazinamide were not done because they are unreliable, experience indicates that M. kansasii is almost always highly resistant to this drug. As soon as these laboratory reports are available, drug treatment should be changed; streptomycin may be used, with either cycloserine or ethionamide as a companion drug, and isoniazid may be continued. If the organisms are resistant to all the antituberculosis drugs, they may be susceptible to one or more of the broad-spectrum antibiotics; cases are known in which the organisms were inhibited by erythromycin, and other antibiotics may sometimes be effective. Any effective drug may be used. If the bacteria are resistant to all known drugs, they should nevertheless be given two-drug therapy, and one of the drugs should be isoniazid. In all cases, drug therapy should be guided by the clinical course of the patient, by the serial x rays, and by the results of laboratory studies. Drug therapy should be continued for two years or longer, but the individual drugs may be changed if progress is unsatisfactory and if alternative drugs are available.

Though chemotherapy is successful in a good percentage of cases, failure to convert sputum and to close cavities is much more common in disease due to unclassified mycobacteria than in tuberculosis. This is understandable, since initial drug resistance is so common with these bacilli. As a result, resectional surgery is needed much more commonly than in the case in tuberculosis. The most common indication for resection is the persistence of cavitation. Here the indication is very strong, since cultures from the resected cavities are very often positive even when the sputum cultures have become negative (10). When disease is due to M. kansasii, resection is necssary to remove residual cavitation in 30 to 50 per cent of cases. Since many patients are still sputum-positive at the time of surgery, there is some additional risk of complications, but this risk is not prohibitive unless there is persistent endobronchitis.

Since there is no evidence that disease due to unclassified mycobacteria is infectious, these patients need not be isolated. Certainly there is no justification for their enforced hospitalization. However, because these diseases are relatively refractory to treatment, and because the required bacteriological studies are rather complex, treatment should be begun in a hospital. Studies in a hospital are almost a necessity, both to establish the diagnosis and to do the drug-susceptibility studies on which intelligent treatment must be based. Not only should treatment be begun in a hospital, but it should be continued in a hospital until the disease is controlled as well as possible by drugs, until a decision has been made as to the need for surgery, and until surgery has been carried out if it is needed. When this has been accomplished, the patient may be discharged and subsequent treatment may be carried out at home, either by his own physician or by an outpatient clinic. It is important to the patient whether he is positive or negative, since this offers some measure of how well he is responding to treatment, but it is not important to the public health. These patients should be treated by drugs for at least two years, and often much longer. They should be observed carefully, for the relapse rate is high, especially in the case of patients with M. kansasii infections.

Case Report

Disease Due to M. Fortuitum. A white man, fifty-seven years of age, noticed cough, expectoration, shortness of breath, weakness, fatigue and anorexia beginning about June 1962, and lost about 30 pounds in weight in the next six months. Early in December 1964, a chest x ray showed bilateral pulmonary disease and sputum was positive for acid-fast bacilli. He was admitted to the Butler Veterans Administration Hospital on December 6, 1962. There examination showed a chronically ill, emaciated man (height 5 feet, 11 inches, weight 103 pounds) with a temperature of 100.2° F. Chest x ray showed that both upper lobes were markedly shrunken and contained multiple cavities. Sputum smears repeatedly showed acid-fast bacilli. On December 13, 1962, he was started on isoniazid, 200 mg three times daily and PAS 4 gm three times daily, with pyridoxine 50 mg three times daily. He did not show any improvement. Susceptibility tests were done on cultures planted on December 11, 1962 and December 13, 1962, and these were reported as follows.

Resistant to isoniazid, 5 μg per ml.
Resistant to streptomycin, 10 μg per ml.
Resistant to PAS, 25 μg per ml.
Resistant to cycloserine, 100 μg per ml.
Resistant to viomycin, 10 μg per ml.
Resistant to penicillin, 10 μg per ml.
Resistant to novobiocin, 30 μg per ml.
Resistant to oleandomycin, 15 μg per ml.
Susceptible to chlortetracycline, 30 μg per ml.
Susceptible to chloramphenicol, 30 μg per ml.
Susceptible to erythromycin, 15 μg per ml.

The organism was catalase positive, neutral red positive, and niacin negative, and was identified as Mycobacterium fortuitum. As a result of these findings, chemotherapy was changed on March 20, 1963, to isoniazid 200 mg three times daily, streptomycin 1 gm daily, and pyrazinamide 1 gm three times daily. On this regimen he gained a little weight and strength, there was slight clearing by x ray, sputum volume diminished, and, most important, the sputum was converted to negative. The last positive culture was planted on May 8, 1963, and the last positive concentrate was obtained on July 10, 1963; subsequent monthly concentrates and cultures were all negative. He was discharged on May 22, 1964. Since then he has taken isoniazid and PAS at home, and has been seen monthly at a State Clinic. There has been no further change in the extensive bilateral cavitary disease, but the sputum has remained negative.

This case is unusual in that M. fortuitum is usually a bacillus of feeble virulence and rarely produces such extensive disease.

Had the patient not responded to the combination of drugs used, chlortetracycline, chloramphenicol and erythormycin were available for trial, since bacteriological tests indicated that the bacillus was susceptible to these drugs. There was no possibility of resectional surgery in this case; it was ruled out by the extent and bilateral nature of the disease and by the severe emphysema.

Case Report

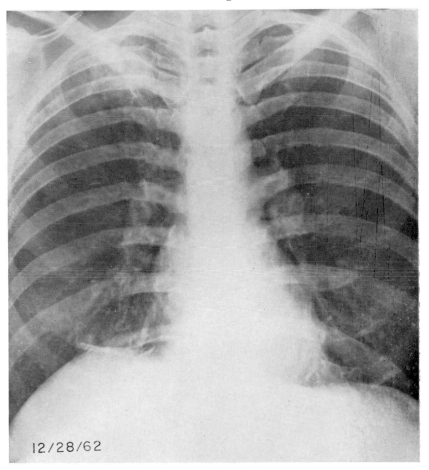

12/28/62

Figure 7

Disease Due to M. Kansasii. A white man, forty-six years of age was found to have pulmonary disease in August, 1962, as a result of a routine chest x ray. He was admitted to a tuberculosis hospital where x rays showed disease in the right upper lobe and sputum concentrates and cultures were repeatedly positive for acid-fast bacilli. The cultures were all described as "pigmented," but the diagnosis of pulmonary tuberculosis was made and the patient was treated with streptomycin and isoniazid. He left the hospital in January, 1963 and discontinued treatment. He was admitted to the Butler Veterans Administration Hospital on February 3, 1964.

At that hospital the chest x ray showed a lesion in the right upper lobe, and planigrams demonstrated a cavity. Sputum concentrates showed acid-fast bacilli. Treatment was started with streptomycin 1 gm twice weekly and isoniazid 100 mg three times daily. Cultures planted on February 5, 1964, March 16, 1964, and April 2, 1964 showed an unusual and consistent drug-susceptibility pattern as follows.

Resistant to isoniazid, 5 μg per ml.
Resistant to streptomycin, 10 μg per ml.
Resistant to PAS, 25 μg per ml.
Resistant to capreomycin, 10μg per ml.
Resistant to viomycin, 10 μg per ml.
Resistant to cycloserine, 5 μg per ml.
Resistant to penicillin, 10 μg per ml.
Susceptible to erythromycin, 15 μg per ml.
Susceptible to chloramphenicol, 30 μg per ml.
Susceptible to tetracycline, 30 μg per ml.
Susceptible to kanamycin, 30 μg per ml.

The organism had a violently positive catalase reaction and was niacin negative and neutral red negative. It was identified as Mycobacterium kansasii.

Cycloserine was added to his therapy on April 20, 1964, and was increased to 250 mg four times daily on April 27, 1964, and pyrazinamide 1 gm three times daily was added on May 1, 1964. On May 5, 1964 his right upper lobe was removed. The resected lobe showed a chronic granulomatous lesion compatible with tuberculosis, and contained foci 1 cm in diameter. Smears were positive for acid-fast bacilli, but cultures from the resected lobe revealed growth characteristics and a drug-resistant pattern identical with that showed by sputum cultures before surgery; the bacilli from the resected specimen were shown to be M. kansasii.

Sputum planted on May 11 and June 2, 1964 still showed M. kansasii on culture. Streptomycin was discontinued, cycloserine was gradually increased to 500 mg four times daily with pyridoxine, and erythromycin 250 mg four times daily was added. Sputum cultures were negative on August 13 and August 27, 1964. The patient gained 15 pounds in weight. He was discharged on October 8, 1964, and is continuing to take isoniazid and erythromycin under the supervision of a State Clinic. All sputum examinations since discharge have been reported negative.

SUMMARY

Disease due to unclassified mycobacteria is being recognized with increasing frequency, and accounts for more than 5 per cent of all admissions to tuberculosis hospitals in some parts of the United States. Most of these infections are due to M. kansasii and the Battey bacillus, but other organisms are also sometimes the cause of disease. Symptoms, x-ray findings, and even histopathological examination of tissue, fail to differentiate these infections from true tuberculosis. The differentiation can be made only by complex laboratory studies in which attention is paid to growth characteristics of the bacilli and their biochemical reactions.

Differentiation is important, since these bacteria are often resistant to many of the antituberculosis drugs. Treatment is based on treatment with two or more effective drugs, often supplemented with resectional surgery. The results of proper treatment are fairly good, though not quite as good as in true tuberculosis. Once maximum benefit has been achieved the patient may be discharged even if his sputum is still positive, since there is no evidence that this type of disease is infectious.

REFERENCES

1. BRANCH, A.: A study of acid-fast organisms other than mammalian tubercle bacilli isolated from disease in man. *Tubercle, 14*:337, 1933.
2. FELDMAN, W. H., DAVIES, R., MOSES, H. E., AND ANDBERG, W.: An unusual mycobacterium isolated from sputum of a man suffering from pulmonary disease of long duration. *Amer. Rev. Tuberc., 48*:82, 1943.
3. RUNYON, E. H.: Anonymous mycobacteria in pulmonary disease. *Med. Clin. N. Amer., 43*:273, 1959.

4. EDWARDS, L. B., AND PALMER, C. E.: Isolation of "atypical" mycobacteria from healthy persons. *Amer. Rev. Resp. Dis., 80*:747,
   1959.

5. TARSHIS, M. S.: The induced development of atypical variants of
   the H37RV strain of M. tuberculosis under the influence of streptomycin and isoniazid *in vitro. Trans. 17th Conference Chemotherapy Tuberculosis,* p. 298, 1958.

6. FELDMAN, W. H., AND AUERBACH, O.: Histopathology of granulomatous lesions associated with Battey-like mycobacteria. *Trans.
   22nd Research Conference Pulmonary Diseases,* p. 239, 1963.

7. CHAPMAN, J. S.: The present status of the unclassified mycobacteria
   (Editorial). *Amer. J. Med., 33*:471, 1962.

8. JENKINS, D. E., BAHAR, D., AND CHOFNAS, I.: Pulmonary disease
   due to atypical mycobacteria. *Trans. 19th Conference Chemotherapy Tuberculosis,* p. 224, 1960.

9. PFUETZE, K. H.: Pulmonary disease caused by the unclassified acid-
   fast bacilli. *Postgrad. Med., 36*:479, 1964.

10. LESTER, W., COLTON, R., AND KENT, G.: Mycobacteria isolated from
    resected lungs. *Amer. Rev. Resp. Dis., 85*:847, 1962.

Chapter XIII

DRUGS IN THE PREVENTION OF
TUBERCULOSIS

The chemoprophylaxis of tuberculosis means the use of the anti-tuberculosis drugs for the prevention rather than the treatment of tuberculosis. There are two varieties, primary and secondary chemoprophylaxis. In the primary variety, one attempts to prevent the infection of people exposed to tubercle bacilli, while in secondary chemoprophylaxis one attempts to prevent the evolution of clinical tuberculosis by people who have already become infected.

For this purpose isoniazid is the ideal drug. It is cheap, it is easy to administer, it is effective against tubercle bacilli when taken by mouth, its toxicity is minimal even when it is taken for long periods of time, and its use does not cause any alteration in the normal microbial flora (1). For prophylaxis, two drugs are not necessary, isoniazid alone being perfectly adequate unless the infecting bacilli are resistant to this drug. Up to the present time, primary isoniazid resistance is not common enough to justify the use of two drugs for prophylaxis.

Primary chemoprophylaxis, that is, the use of isoniazid to prevent tuberculous infection in people who are heavily exposed but tuberculin negative, is still controversial, but most believe that it has a place in situations involving high risk. Such situations may occur when uninfected infants live in close contact with patients with open tuberculosis, or when a laboratory worker accidentally inoculates himself with large numbers of tubercle bacilli as a result of plunging a contaminated needle into a finger. Primary prophylaxis seems to be beneficial in such situations. A United States Public Health Service study has shown that this type of prophylaxis is successful in preventing primary tuberculosis in children living in households with people who have open tuberculosis (2). However, in such cases isoniazid protects only so long as it is taken, and when it is stopped the child is as susceptible to infection as before.

In the case of a tuberculin-negative child exposed to tuberculosis in the home, isoniazid prophylaxis need not be continued very long if the child is separated from the source of infection. This child, having been removed from the source of infection, should receive isoniazid as prophylaxis, to prevent the development of a primary infection from the tubercle bacilli he may have already acquired. Since the administration of isoniazid early in the latent period of primary tuberculosis prolongs the latent period, and since it is desired to continue prophylaxis until the latent period is over, isoniazid should be continued for about four months. At the end of that time, if the child is still tuberculin-negative, he should receive BCG vaccine to provide immunity. Another plan is to vaccinate him with BCG while he is still receiving isoniazid prophylaxis. Since isoniazid will inhibit the growth of the modified tubercle bacilli which constitutes BCG, either large doses of BCG must be given or one must use an isoniazid-resistant BCG. An isoniazid-resistant BCG is available, and it is as effective as standard BCG in producing immunity. BCG is preferable to primary chemoprophylaxis for the protection of tuberculin-negative medical students, nurses or others who may expect heavy exposure to tuberculosis in the future (3). In the case of a laboratory accident in which tubercle bacilli are inoculated, isoniazid should be started at once.

There is one theoretical objection to primary prophylaxis. By giving isoniazid prophylactically, one may not only prevent the growth and multiplication of any tubercle bacilli which may have been acquired, which is desirable, but may also prevent the development of immunity to tuberculosis, which is undesirable. If the tubercle bacilli are eradicated by isoniazid this does not matter, but if some bacilli survive they would be able to resume growth after isoniazid is stopped, and then the absence of immunity would be a liability. It is for this reason that BCG vaccination is recommended along with primary isoniazid prophylaxis.

In secondary chemoprophylaxis, that is, when isoniazid is given with the intention of preventing the development of disease after infection has already taken place and the tuberculin test has already become positive, this theoretical objection does not exist. It is true that full immunity has not yet evolved at the time the tuberculin test first becomes positive; tuberculin sensitivity develops a little earlier than the peak of acquired immunity. This is not a significant objection, however. Chemoprophylaxis is usually started at some time after the skin sensitivity has become positive. Even if it is begun at the exact moment the skin sensitivity becomes positive, there is already a substantial degree of acquired immunity. Besides, to the person recently infected with tuberculosis, isoniazid offers a much greater degree of protection than acquired immunity; in spite of acquired immunity a significant number of people develop progressive tuberculosis, while those who receive isoniazid chemoprophylaxis seldom develop active disease.

Another theoretical objection has been raised to secondary chemoprophylaxis. It has been speculated that as a result of the exposure of the tubercle bacilli to isoniazid they might develop resistance to this drug. There is very little risk of resistance developing in this situation. In order for resistance to develop, it is necessary to have large numbers of actively multiplying tubercle bacilli exposed to the drug. This permits the emergence of drug-resistant mutants, and then the administration of the drug suppresses the susceptible bacilli but permits the growth of resistant bacilli. However, in a latent infection there is no cavity, the number of tubercle bacilli is small, and the bacilli are not multiplying rapidly, so the administration of isoniazid is unlikely to result in the appearance of drug-resistant strains. This may happen occasionally, but it is such a rare occurrence that it should not discourage the use of isoniazid in prophylaxis.

There has been some concern about the possible toxicity of isoniazid used for a year prophylactically. Isoniazid, however, is a drug of very low toxicity. Peripheral neuritis is the only toxic manifestation that occurs with any frequency, and even this is uncommon in children. Certainly the fear of toxicity need not deter anyone from using this drug prophylactically.

There are practical problems involved in the use of isoniazid in the prophylaxis of tuberculosis. It is difficult to be sure that the isoniazid tablets are actually taken, and it is costly and troublesome to administer extensive prophylactic programs. For instance, in the

United States Public Health Service trials among household contacts, 25,000 children were followed for a year. About a third of these persons failed to take their tablets regularly, and about a tenth took them sporadically or not at all. In this study seventy-eight persons in the untreated group developed significant tuberculosis during the year of the study, as contrasted with only eighteen in the treated group (2). An expensive program had to be organized, isoniazid tablets had to be provided for 12,500 children, and a follow-up of these children had to be developed, in order to prevent sixty cases of active tuberculosis. Furthermore, there is reason to suspect that a few of these sixty children had their tuberculosis postponed rather than prevented, since it is known that tubercle bacilli are seldom eradicated by chemoprophylaxis, and those organisms which survive may cause disease later (4). Yet chemoprophylaxis seems worthwhile. In the study just mentioned, sixty cases of tuberculosis were prevented, most of them permanently. The prevention of disease is one of the most worthwhile aspects of medicine.

Recent tuberculous infection without evidence of clinical disease is the strongest indication for chemoprophylaxis. Much serious dissemination of tuberculosis takes place within the first year or so after infection. Eighty-five per cent of nurses who developed a positive tuberculin reaction and later developed lesions of active tuberculosis did so within two years of infection. For this reason it is wise to give isoniazid to those who have recently been infected (5). Children under the age of three may be regarded as having been infected recently if they have a positive tuberculin reaction, and so should receive chemoprophylaxis. Older children or adults who are known to have developed a positive tuberculin reaction within a year also fall within this group. More controversial is the question of prophylaxis of adults or older children who have a positive tuberculin reaction, but whose date of conversion is unknown. The mere existence of a positive tuberculin reaction of unknown duration does not justify the use of isoniazid in these people. However, if the reaction is large (15 mm or more induration after testing with 5 T. U. of PPD), this is often an indication of either recent infection or of the presence of some degree of activity, and therefore chemoprophylaxis is justified. This is particularly true in children in the teens, when the risk of developing active tuberculosis is markedly increased in the group with large tuberculin reactions.

Tuberculous infection without manifest disease, evidenced only by a positive reaction, is not in itself a reason for chemoprophylaxis. However, there are a number of situations in which the patient is more vulnerable than most people to tuberculosis, and in these situations chemoprophylaxis should be advised. First to be considered are teen-aged children, especially girls, who have a positive tuberculin re-action. In these children it is known that the risk of development of active tuberculosis is quite high, especially if the reaction is of large size, so it is desirable to use chemoprophylaxis to protect them. Second is the group of patients who are to receive long-term adreno-corticosteroid therapy—for rheumatoid arthritis, perhaps. It is im-portant to know if these patients have been infected with tuberculosis before steroids are started. If the tuberculin reaction is positive, the individual should receive isoniazid prophylaxis for the entire duration of steroid hormone therapy and for three months longer. By reducing the body defenses against infection, the steroids are capable of caus-ing a disastrous spread of disease from the smallest tuberculous focus, even from a focus which cannot be demonstrated by x-ray. For this reason isoniazid prophylaxis is mandatory when a positive tuberculin reaction exists in a patient who is scheduled to receive long-term steroid therapy. It is necessary that the tuberculin test be done be-fore steroid therapy is begun; after steroids have been administered the tuberculin test is no longer reliable, since these hormones are capable of suppressing a positive reaction.

Case Report

This white man first noticed joint pain in the right hand in 1956 when he was forty-four years old. The diagnosis of rheuma-toid arthritis was made, and treatment was started with aspirin and physical therapy. Since this did not control his pain, steroid therapy was begun in 1957. At that time chest x ray was negative but tuberculin reaction was positive. He received prednisone 5 mg four times daily, at first in a hospital and later as an out-patient, until March, 1962. At that time an attempt was made to reduce the steroid dosage, but fever developed at once. Prednisolone was substituted for prednisone, however. In spite of treatment the arthritis progressed relentlessly, so that by 1962 both hands and wrists were deformed, crippled and painful, the right femoral head was completely destroyed, there was involvement of both knees, ankles and left shoulder, and there were florid rheumatoid nodules on both arms. He complained also of weakness and weight loss. X ray of the chest showed pulmonary tuberculosis, so he was admitted to the hospital on August 7, 1962.

On admission he was acutely ill, with a fever of 103° F. Chest x ray showed a very extensive lesion involving all lobes of both lungs, with multiple cavities. Sputum was positive for acid-fast bacilli on smear and culture.

This case illustrates the risk of using steroid hormones without the simultaneous use of isoniazid. This patient had no evidence of pulmonary tuberculosis when steroid therapy was begun, but he did have a positive tuberculin reaction. The use of isoniazid concurrently would probably have prevented the development of this tuberculous lesion.

Another situation in which isoniazid prophylaxis is justified is in tuberculin-positive children who are suffering from a severe, debilitating illness (6). Their resistance to tuberculosis is diminished thereby, and their risk of developing the disease is therefore increased. In this situation it is desirable to give isoniazid throughout the illness and for three months thereafter.

Primary tuberculosis, with lesions visible by x ray and a history of the recent development of a positive tuberculin reaction, is a strong indication for chemoprophylaxis. Sometimes this hastens the resolution of the primary complex, but even if it does not it is almost always effective in preventing the dissemination of tubercle bacilli from this complex, and it is likely that it will prevent the development of later lesions of active tuberculosis.

Case Report

At the age of twenty-one this nurse began her duties on a surgical ward. A majority of the patients in her care had thoracic surgery, and in about half of the cases the surgery was done for pulmonary tuberculosis. Her tuberculin reaction was negative when she came on duty on October 23, 1961, and remained negative for nearly three years. Tests done on April 16, 1962, October 8, 1962, May 22, 1963, November 6, 1963 and June 22, 1964 were all negative. On December 14, 1964 the tuberculin reaction was strongly positive (15 mm induration to PPD intermediate). There was no other evidence of tuberculous disease—no fever, no cough or sputum, no x ray evidence of infiltration, and several gastric cultures were negative.

On December 20, 1964, chemoprophylaxis was started, employing 100 mg isoniazid three times daily, with the intention of continuing this medication for a year. This use of the drug is of course not expected to bring about symptomatic improvement or x-ray clearing, because no symptoms or x-ray findings exist. The purpose of chemoprophylaxis is to prevent the progression of the primary lesion locally, or the dissemination of tuberculosis from the primary focus.

Inactive pulmonary tuberculosis is attended by a small but significant risk of reactivation. Increasingly, active cases of tuberculosis are coming from individuals who were infected in the past rather than from those infected recently (7). There are circumstances in which the risk can be greatly reduced by isoniazid prophylaxis. If the tuberculosis has become inactive as a result of treatment which either did not include chemotherapy or which included a course of chemotherapy which is now believed to be inadequate, a course of chemoprophylaxis is desirable. Studies have shown that the frequency of reactivation in such cases is reduced by isoniazid prophylaxis.

If a pulmonary lesion is found on a routine chest x ray and it is believed to be tuberculosis, but there is neither clinical nor bacteriological evidence that the disease is active, a course of chemoprophylaxis is likewise desirable. In this situation every effort must be made to establish a definite diagnosis before starting isoniazid. This is not because there is any risk in giving isoniazid unnecessarily. The risk is rather in missing the correct diagnosis in our anxiety to prevent tuberculosis, so that isoniazid is given for tuberculosis when actually there is another disease which requires treatment. There are some conditions which lower the patient's resistance to tuberculosis; such conditions are the post-gastrectomy state, diabetes, pneumonia, silicosis, chronic malnutrition or the prolonged administration of corticosteroid drugs. If any of these conditions co-exist with inactive pulmonary tuberculosis, a course of isoniazid prophylaxis is justified (6).

Pregnancy does not favor the development of tuberculosis, but childbearing and the puerperium are attended by some risk of re-activation of this disease; therefore during this period patients with inactive tuberculosis should receive chemoprophylaxis. When isoniazid prophylaxis is planned in the case of significant though inactive pulmonary tuberculosis, close supervision is necessary for the entire period of prophylaxis (8). This is necessary to assure that the isoniazid is being taken regularly, that there is no progression of the lesion by x ray, and that the sputum remains negative. If there is clinical or radiological evidence of activity or if the sputum is found to be positive, single-drug prophylaxis is no longer adequate, and an effective two-drug program of therapy must replace it.

Case Report

In 1947 this man, then 20 years of age, was found by routine chest x-ray to have a small lesion in the 2nd anterior interspace on the left. This lesion was compatible with minimal pulmonary tuberculosis. The patient had no symptoms at all—no cough, expectoration, weakness, weight loss or fever. His tuberculin reaction was positive to first strength PPD, and gastric culture was positive for acid-fast bacilli on two occasions. He was admitted to the hospital on April 7, 1947. He received no antituberculosis drugs, and since no cavity was ever demonstrated he received no collapse therapy, but was treated by bedrest. The lesion slowly regressed, and gastric culture was last positive on June 10, 1947. He was discharged on November 12, 1947, and several months later he returned to work. He has remained well.

In 1960 it was recommended that, since he had proven inactive pulmonary tuberculosis and had never had chemotherapy, it would be prudent for him to take chemoprophylaxis. Consequently he took isoniazid 100 mg 3 times daily for one year, without any other change in his way of life. He is still working and has remained well.

The recommended prophylactic dose of isoniazid for adults and older children is 300 mg daily and for young children 8 to 10 mg per kg body weight. This may be given in a single daily dose or in divided doses. Chemoprophylaxis should in general be continued for one year.

Thus far in this chapter we have spoken only of drugs used specifically for the prevention of tuberculosis—the prevention of the infection itself, the prevention of the evolution of a primary infection into clinical disease, and the prevention of reactivation of inactive tuberculosis. But drugs used for the treatment of tuberculosis rapidly reduce sputum volume and infectivity, making the treated patient far less dangerous to his family, his friends, his community and the personnel who take care of him at home or in the hospital. By thus reducing the infectivity of the patient with active tuberculosis, the source of all infection, drugs used primarily for treatment really perform an important function in prevention. Drugs used for the treatment of tuberculosis, therefore, also play an important role in prevention (7).

SUMMARY

The use of isoniazid to prevent tuberculosis has much to recommend it. The drug is effective against tubercle bacilli, cheap and easy to take. It is of very low toxicity, and does not cause any alteration in the normal bacterial flora. The indications for its prophylactic use are limited, but in these situations it may do a great deal of good. The principal indications for its use are the following.

1. Heavy exposure to tuberculosis, even though still tuberculin negative.
   a. Infants.
   b. Young children.
2. Recent tuberculous infection without manifest clinical disease.
   a. Children under age 3 with positive tuberculin reaction.
   b. Adults or older children who have developed a positive tuberculin reaction within a year.
3. Tuberculous infection, manifested by a positive tuberculin reaction, in patients receiving long-term steroid therapy.
4. Tuberculin positive children during serious chronic illness.
5. Inactive tuberculosis—special situations.
   a. No previous chemotherapy.
   b. Inadequate previous chemotherapy.
   c. Co-existing conditions which lower host resistance or otherwise threaten to cause reactivation of tuberculosis.
      (1) Diabetes mellitus.

(2) Silicosis.
(3) Pneumonia.
(4) Post-gastrectomy state.
(5) Pregnancy.

REFERENCES

1. McDermott, W., Raffel, S., Canetti, G., Holm, J., Lincoln, E. M., Schmidt, L. H., and Youmans, G. P.: Chemoprophylaxis of tuberculosis. *Amer. Rev. Resp. Dis., 80:, Part 2:*1, 1959.
2. Ferebee, S. H., and Mount, F. W.: Tuberculosis morbidity in a controlled trial of the prophylactic use of isoniazid among household contacts. *Amer. Rev. Resp. Dis., 85:*490, 1962.
3. Canetti, G.: The eradication of tuberculosis. Theoretical problems and practical solutions. *Tubercle, 43:*300, 1962.
4. McDermott, W.: Drug-microbe-host mechanisms involved in a consideration of chemoprophylaxis. *Bull. Int. Un. Tuberc., 29:*243, 1959.
5. Lambert, H. P.: The chemoprophylaxis of tuberculosis. *Amer. Rev. Resp. Dis., 80:*648, 1959.
6. Zorini, A. O.: Further development in human and bovine antituberculosis chemoprophylaxis with isoniazid in Italy. *Dis. Chest, 43:*131, 1963.
7. Arden House Conference on Tuberculosis, Public Health Service Publication No. 784, 1961.
8. Chaves, A. D.: Pulmonary tuberculosis. *Mod. Treat., 1:*330, 1964.

INDEX